Eat to Beat Arthritis

Over 60 ... a self-treatment plan to transform your life

Marguerite Patten, O.B.E. *and*

Jeannette Ewin, Ph.D.

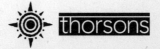

Thorsons
An Imprint of HarperCollins*Publishers*
77–85 Fulham Palace Road
Hammersmith, London W6 8JB

The website address is: www.thorsonselement.com

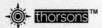 ™

and *Thorsons* are trademarks of
HarperCollins*Publishers* Limited

First published by Thorsons 2001
This edition 2004

10 9 8 7 6 5 4 3 2 1

A catalogue record for this book
is available from the British Library

ISBN 0 00 716966 3

Printed and bound in Great Britain by
Clays Ltd, St Ives plc

Eat to Beat Arthritis

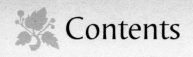

Contents

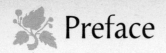 # Preface

Marguerite Patten, O.B.E., a well-known and highly respected food writer, and Jeannette Ewin, Ph.D., a health journalist with an international following, have joined forces to create an eating plan that can help you beat the pain and distress of arthritis. The *Eat to Beat Arthritis* Diet, and everything you need to know about how it can change your life, is contained in this book.

Arthritis has been compared to being locked in a prison: its symptoms bar you from living the way you wish. In this book you will learn how to break lifestyle habits that have shackled you to pain. The pages that follow contain the latest information about food supplements that fight the causes and symptoms of arthritis. You will also learn how to listen to your own body, and understand what it is telling you about the food you eat.

The *Eat to Beat Arthritis* Diet is based on a selection of foods and supplements that help your body fight the pain of crippling disease. Unlike other diets you may have tried in the past, it allows you to enjoy appetizing and satisfying meals while you chart the dietary course towards wellbeing. Using foods recommended in the *Eat to Beat Arthritis* Diet, Marguerite Patten has developed over 60 delicious recipes that can be enjoyed by everyone – not just those suffering from arthritis. Unlike the recipes you may have tried in some health-related cookery books, the dishes described here are full of appealing flavour and texture.

Working on this book was a labour of love for Marguerite, as she personally knows how arthritis can affect one's life. Her search for a means of controlling this painful illness had been long and hard, and included both acupuncture and chiropractic treatments. When these failed, her doctor said surgery on a severely arthritic hip was the only answer. Faced with family and professional responsibilities, Marguerite's response was, 'Sorry. I haven't the time right now.' With hope of finding an answer to her advancing illness in some other form of therapy, she turned for help to the subject she knows best: food. By changing her diet she changed her life, and in this book she not only provides clear instructions about how to cook the appropriate foods, but also shares the secrets of her own story.

Reading every health and diet book she could find that focused on the perplexing problem of arthritis, Marguerite came across an international bestseller: *A Doctor's Proven New Home Cure for Arthritis*, by Dr Giraud W. Campbell. Here was a healing diet that incorporated foods she enjoyed eating. The prescribed therapy was strict, but manageable. She gave it a try and within weeks experienced a dramatic and clinically recognizable improvement in her condition.

Over the years since her introduction to Dr Campbell's book, much has been learned about how diets work and why certain nutrient supplements help control this debilitating illness. To share her personal experience, and to expand what she had learned about diet and arthritis, Marguerite Patten teamed up with a friend and nutritionist, Dr Jeannette Ewin. Taking their lead from Dr Campbell's book, they developed the *Eat to Beat Arthritis* Diet. This sensible and healthy way to enjoy good food combines Marguerite's decades of experience developing tasty and sure-fire recipes, with Jeannette's insight into the interactions between food, nutrition and health. As a side benefit, those who follow their advice will soon find they not only gain control over pain, but also enjoy a greater feeling of wellbeing.

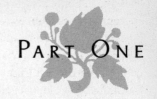

PART ONE

You Can Beat Arthritis!

Chapter 1

You can beat arthritis!

During an awards ceremony, American comedian Jack Benny reportedly said: 'Thank you for this honour, but I don't know what I did to deserve it. Then again, I have arthritis, and I don't know what I did to deserve that either.'

If – like Jack Benny – you suffer from arthritis, you know it is no laughing matter. Pain can dominate your life, and its effects are insidious. You don't sleep well at night because your joints hurt. Backache plagues you while you are in bed. Knees and hips ache when you get out of bed. Slowly, you begin to feel depressed by the lack of sleep. During the day you begin avoiding exercise. Taking a walk, swinging a golf club, or doing everyday household chores cause discomfort and pain and, as a result, you find yourself moving less. Muscles that were once firm and strong begin to weaken from lack of use. Not burning off calories as quickly as you once did, you find yourself gaining a bit of weight. The problem of wakeful nights becomes compounded because the exercise you now avoid is an important part of getting the body ready for sleep. Over time, arthritis begins to dominate your life, and you find yourself in a slow physical and emotional cycle of decline.

The above scenario is not inevitable, however. You can prevent it happening to you. By changing your diet and lifestyle, it is possible to regain a sense of physical and mental wellbeing. Arthritis leads to negative changes in your life: The *Eat to Beat Arthritis* Diet is your guide to the positive changes needed to overcome them.

Unfortunately, many arthritis sufferers never find a way of overcoming the debilitating symptoms of the disease. They may seek help from their doctor, and find that the medication they are prescribed causes unpleasant side effects such as stomach pain. Others try various forms of alternative therapy only to find them ineffective. In the end, they all too often submit. After all, they may reason, everyone who reaches a certain age must suffer from some form of aches or pains. As time goes by, their condition gets worse. All too soon the activities they once enjoyed – like playing with the grandchildren, gardening, or keeping up with a favourite hobby – cause too much pain to bear.

Don't give in to arthritis. By learning to select and enjoy the foods that uniquely suit you, and by following the lifestyle advice in this book, you can continue enjoying life. Think positive. Be positive. Make the changes that release you from the negative cycle of arthritis.

The *Eat to Beat Arthritis* Diet is based on a simple, three-part strategy to healing and health:

* Know your enemy (in this case – arthritis);
* Know how to defeat your enemy (gain control over arthritis in seven weeks); and
* Enjoy life.

The details of this strategy are outlined in the chapters that follow, but here is a brief summary of what is involved.

Know your enemy

Strip away the mystery of arthritis by understanding what it is and why it occurs. When an illness is diagnosed and given a name by a doctor, it has power. It is the unknown, and we are its victims. By learning something about an illness, or disease, and why it makes us suffer, we gain control. Knowledge replaces doubt, and hope replaces fear.

The basic facts outlined in Chapter 2 demystify arthritis. More detailed information is presented in the section of the book called 'Questions and answers about arthritis'. Additional help is also provided by a glossary, a selection of good food tips and a list of helpful resources (this includes a number of websites for those of you with access to the internet).

Know how to defeat your enemy
(gain control over arthritis in seven weeks)

This book is your guide to seven weeks that can change your life. Once you understand an illness, you can build a strategy to defeat it. If its total defeat is not possible, you can still find ways to minimize its symptoms and learn to live a brighter, fuller life.

In the early parts of this book you will learn how to alter your diet and lifestyle to break the negative cycle of arthritis. You will discover why good nutrition can rebuild failing tissues, block pain and revitalize aching joints. It will also become clear why certain foods should be avoided, and how everyday favourites – like tomatoes and aubergines (eggplants) – can cause joint pain and swelling.

You are unique, and your requirement for food is unique. Not only do you need to know which foods you should eat, but how they can be balanced to help you live a full and active life – despite having arthritis. This is explained in Chapter 3, where you will find an outline of the basic rules of nutrition, and information about how the substances in food affect your health. The basic rules of nutrition hold for everyone, but the amounts of individual nutrients you require for optimum health are not the same as those needed by others.

During the seven weeks of this diet, you will learn how to listen to your body and recognize when specific foods are doing harm. Simply by avoiding all foods containing wheat and all drinks containing caffeine, many arthritis suffers find their lives changed forever.

If all this is beginning to sound a bit too restrictive – take heart! In Part Two you will find a long list of foods you *can* eat. And to help you enjoy a delicious (and very modern) approach to cooking with these ingredients, Marguerite Patten has devised over 60 easy-to-prepare recipes.

Marguerite's recipes are a vital part of this book. In them she not only explains what to cook and how, but also shares her own experience with the diet. Day by day, step by step, she takes you through the diet and discusses why she chose one ingredient over another. These personal insights give invaluable information and encouragement as you begin to experiment with a style of cooking that is fresh and tasty as well as healing and healthy.

Enjoy life

This is the third proclamation of the *Eat to Beat Arthritis* Diet. Unfortunately there are no simple recipes to help you with this part of the programme. Some suggestions are offered later on, but no one can prescribe what is best for *you*. Just remember:

* The glass of life is half full – *not* half empty.
* Smiling has been scientifically shown to have a positive effect on mood and the sensation of pain.
* Exercise relaxes you, loosens joints and muscles, and helps lay the groundwork for a good night's sleep.

CHAPTER 2

Know your enemy

(understanding arthritis and its causes)

The costly epidemic of arthritis

'People ignore arthritis both as public and personal health problems because it doesn't kill you.' So said Chad Helmick, a medical epidemiologist at the Center for Disease Control and Prevention in the United States. He continued: 'But what they don't realize is that as Americans work and live longer, arthritis can affect their quality of life and eventually lead to disability.' According to the *FDA Consumer* (May–June 2000), who quoted Dr Helmick, the current annual cost of arthritis to the U.S. economy is nearly $65 billion – a sum large enough to have about the same impact as a moderate recession.

Arthritis can strike at any age, and the number of arthritis sufferers increases each year. During a person's lifetime, arthritis is more likely to restrict activity than cancer, diabetes or heart disease. World-wide, arthritis inflicts a terrible cost. In the United States alone, currently about 42 million people are afflicted by chronic forms of arthritis: according to the Center for Disease Control, that number will rise to 60 million by 2020. More than 11 million of those people will be crippled badly enough to be classified as disabled. And the U.S. is not an exceptional case – the social and economic impact of arthritis in the United States is mirrored throughout the Western world.

Why should more people suffer from arthritis today than in the past? And why do various forms of arthritis appear to be increasing at a greater rate in Westernized countries than in the rest of the world? Many experts believe the answer must be related to our lifestyle and diet.

When you consider the vast amount of money spent on medication to treat the symptoms of arthritis, and on surgical repair of crippled hips and knees, you get some idea just how much could be saved if people would eat and live according to the simple rules suggested here.

Arthritis comes in many forms

The word 'arthritis' refers to any process that causes inflammation of joints and surrounding tissues. Depending on which expert you believe, there are between one and two hundred different conditions that can be classified as 'arthritis'. Some of these are common (osteoarthritis, rheumatoid arthritis and gout), while others are relatively rare (ankylosing spondylitis and systemic lupus erythematosis are examples). In *Eat to Beat Arthritis* we focus on those types of arthritis that affect the most people, although the anti-inflammation diet described here will help almost everyone.

Two key words need explanation: 'inflammation' and 'joint'.

Inflammation is a natural process in which the body's immune system reacts to infection, injury or any abnormal form of irritation. The area of inflammation becomes red, swollen and abnormally warm. When inflammation takes place around a site of infection or injury its role is to kill any invading organisms and speed up the removal of debris from dead bacteria (or viruses) and tissue. In other words, inflammation is a healthy part of the normal healing process. Unfortunately, there are times when the immune system mistakes the body's own normal tissues for the 'enemy', and attacks them. This is known as an auto-immune reaction. The immune system may also attack parts of the body where concentrations of abnormal substances occur – such as joints in which bony nodules form after injury; or in places where abnormal deposits of uric acid form, as is the case in gout.

Inflammation is the real culprit in arthritis, so the diet described in this book is designed to help control inflammation. Even if you are on medication for your condition, changing the way you eat will help break the painful bonds of inflamed joints and tissues.

A *joint* is a place, or 'join', in the body where bones meet. Some joints are stationary, or fused, and have no motion; the joints between

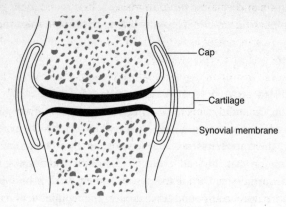

Articular joint

bone in the skull are examples. Other joints may allow a limited degree of motion, such as those in the fingers and toes, while others allow extensive motion. Hip joints are a good example of a place where there can be considerable movement at the place where bones meet.

As a general rule joints are formed from fibrous tissue, a pad of cartilage at the end of each bone within the joint, a thin lining of synovial membrane (which secretes a thin lubricating fluid into the joint to aid its motion) and, sometimes, a ligament, or strong band of fibrous tissue binding the bones together. Ligaments are also found supporting other parts of the body, including some internal organs.

OSTEOARTHRITIS

Almost everyone suffers from some degree of osteoarthritis. The older you get the more likely it is that injury or constant use has damaged one or more of your joints, and osteoarthritis has set in. Many athletes suffer this form of arthritis at a fairly early age owing to injury to cartilage and the bones within much-used joints, such as the knee. In less athletic people the pain experienced in knees, hands and hips by the time they reach retirement age is as a result of simple wear and tear on the internal structure of joints. In both cases, cartilage can wear so thin the ends of bones become exposed within joints. This causes pain and inflammation. To make matters worse, bony nodules may collect in osteoarthritic joints, adding to the pain and inflammation. And as anyone who suffers from pain knows, it can be mentally exhausting as well as physically debilitating.

Medical treatment for osteoarthritis usually involves analgesics (painkillers) and – in some cases – drugs that support the body's attempts to rebuild damaged cartilage. Most of these drugs not only effectively reduce pain, they also reduce inflammation. The problem is that many analgesics (including aspirin and ibuprofen) cause stomach irritation that can lead to bleeding, and they do nothing to help rebuild worn tissue. During the past decade research has shown that there are natural compounds that support the rebuilding of damaged cartilage: *glucosamine* holds the greatest promise at present. You can learn more about this healing compound on page 237.

RHEUMATOID ARTHRITIS

The stiffness, pain, swelling and loss of function associated with rheumatoid arthritis results from inflammation of the lining that secretes lubricating fluid into joints. The disease can affect other parts of the body, but treatment is most often sought for the condition when it involves joints. In most cases this form of arthritis affects the same joint on both sides of the body: both knees, or both hips, or the knuckles of both forefingers. In severe cases deformity and loss of function result.

The medications used to treat rheumatoid and osteoarthritis are similar, and are selected to block pain and reduce inflammation. However, there is strong evidence that certain foods, such as oily fish, and food supplements, such as fish oil, help reduce the causes of the inflammation without endangering the delicate lining of the stomach.

More information about rheumatoid arthritis can be found on page 233.

GOUT

Gout is frequently lampooned as a rich man's illness, associated with too much fine wine and fatty food. In fact it strikes people from all walks of life: beggar and king. It can be very painful, and it is common to hear sufferers describe how they cannot bear to have even the weight of a bed-sheet rest on an affected toe. (Big toes are frequent victims of this illness.) Mercifully, gout is far less common than either osteoarthritis or rheumatoid arthritis.

Gout is caused when too much uric acid collects in the blood. Uric acid is a by-product of normal metabolism, and it is usually collected and discarded from the body by the kidneys in urine. However, when the kidneys are not functioning normally, or when the diet contains an excess of certain foods, blood levels can rise to the point where the excess uric acid crystallizes in joints, the kidneys, or even the soft tissue of the ear. These stone-like residues cause pain, damage surrounding tissues, and trigger the biological processes that lead to inflammation.

There are medications to help gout suffers, but diet is a vital part of controlling the build-up of uric acid in the blood, and reducing or eliminating inflammation.

For more about gout, see page 233.

CHAPTER 3

Know how to combat your enemy

(seven weeks that will change your life)

The power to heal is within you. Given the right nutritional building blocks, adequate rest, exercise and a pollution-free environment, the human body has remarkable powers of restoration and self-healing. The *Eat to Beat Arthritis* Diet is all about harnessing these elements to your advantage.

Food is the answer

No diet should promise overnight success. Healing takes time. If you suffer from arthritis you need to eat foods, and take food supplements, that calm the inflammatory processes that cause pain. You also need to consume those nutrients that the body needs to build new and healthy tissues, such as cartilage in joints.

Think of it this way. Your body is made entirely of the foods you eat. In an ideal world, what you eat would exactly match what your body needs to function at its best. But this is not an ideal world. Stress, illness, lifestyle changes and the natural processes of bearing children all place demands on your body that require a specific blend of nutrients. For example, smoking increases the body's need for vitamin C, and you can cope with stress better if your diet is rich in foods containing B vitamins.

Using the advice in this book you will learn how to select those foods that provide the unique blend of nutrients your body needs for healing. You will also learn how the right foods can help you combat damaging and painful inflammation. Also highlighted is the importance of identifying foods to which you may be sensitive. Once you know what are the right foods for you, you can then go on to prepare delicious dishes using these ingredients. Best of all, you can read Marguerite Patten's excellent advice on using and living with this diet. When you know what suits your body best, and you have experienced the rewards from changing your eating habits to improve your arthritis, you will find that you can relax from time to time and allow yourself some flexibility in what you eat. Marguerite explains how she balances her lifestyle with the diet and allows herself the occasional treat. The trick is just to enjoy yourself, then reinstate the *Eat to Beat Arthritis* Diet as soon as you can afterwards and you'll soon be back to your best.

A schedule for success

Once you begin this diet you will probably experience an improvement in your condition during the first week: but there is more to come! Give yourself at least six weeks before you judge its total benefits to you. Eating plans that promise much faster results are not really being fair. It takes time for your body to heal. The full programme is explained in the next section, but here is a brief week-by-week summary of the diet, followed by an explanation of how it works:

Week zero – *Listening to your body*

* Learn about yourself by keeping records of what you eat and when your symptoms appear.
* As the first step towards controlling pain, eliminate coffee, cola drinks, tea and other sources of caffeine from your diet.
* If you smoke cigarettes, this is the time to stop.

Week one – *Cleansing and detoxifying your body*

* After a one-day fast, begin a diet of foods that help heal and rebuild the body.

- ✳ Eliminate all foods containing wheat, rye, oats, and all sources of gluten from your diet.
- ✳ Eliminate alcohol from your diet.
- ✳ Supplements containing fish oil and vitamin E are added to your healing routine, as is a Health Drink that you make at home.

Week two – *Stabilizing your body*

- ✳ The routine of foods and supplements started during Week One continues. (By this time, many people experience significant relief from the pain and inflammation of arthritis.)

Weeks three through six – *The elimination diet*

- ✳ During these four weeks, you will introduce various foods and food groups into your diet to test their effect on your arthritis.
- ✳ Up to now you have enjoyed a diet based on a limited number of ingredients. To live in the real world of work and family, that list of foods needs to be expanded.
- ✳ The benefits of the diet by now include a greater sense of wellbeing, and improved skin and hair texture.

Week seven and forever – *Enjoy life*

WEEK ZERO – GETTING TO KNOW YOURSELF

This period is a preparation for the life-changes to come. By keeping a daily chart of when and where you experience pain, what you eat, how well you sleep, and when and how you exercise, you will have a snapshot of how well you are taking care of your body. Make no changes during this week (with the exception of giving up caffeine). Just listen to your body. You will continue to keep these charts throughout the first six weeks of the diet, because they will provide information about how your body is reacting to change.

It may be tempting to skip this week's activities. Forget any such ideas. This may be the most valuable week of the diet, because it provides the information you need to monitor your progress towards a life of less pain and greater mobility. Keeping notes for anything shorter than a week will give you a false picture, because your life activities have a pattern – and they run from Sunday through to Saturday.

If you smoke, use this time to consider how you plan to remove this pollutant from your body. As you will learn in the next chapter, smoking adds to the problems that increase the pain of arthritis.

Week one – Cleansing and detoxifying your body
Work begins here. During these seven days you will lower the level of harmful substances in the body through fasting, avoiding specific foods, and drinking adequate amounts of fluids. The charts you keep will begin to show early benefits of the diet.

Week two – Stabilizing your body
By the end of Week One you will be eating a very healthy, although somewhat restricted diet. This is the Basic Arthritis Diet. By following the same eating plan during the second week of the diet, you will stabilize your metabolism and remove any traces of reaction from foods you have eaten in the past. You are allowing your body to rest. (Do not worry about having to eat bland and uninteresting food – the recipes Marguerite Patten provides further on in the book are full of flavour.)

Weeks three to six – Expanding your food vocabulary
Now is the time to expand the variety of foods you eat. In this section, guidance is provided on how to test specific foods for their effect on your level of joint pain and discomfort. You may be surprised by the results. Foods you have enjoyed for years – and that you have been told are good for you – may be just the ones that stimulate an inflammatory reaction in your joints.

WEEK SEVEN AND FOREVER –
HOW TO LIVE A LITTLE AND STILL MAINTAIN CONTROL OVER PAIN

Once you know which foods present problems, and how to detoxify your body on the Basic Arthritis Diet, you can try breaking the rules. But remember: once you break the rules you must return to them as quickly as possible.

CHAPTER 4

Changing your lifestyle

As you change your diet, and learn about yourself by using a self-assessment chart, you should consider other ways to improve your health. In addition to changing your diet and giving up smoking (see box below), there are other ways you can change your lifestyle and help control the painful and crippling effects of arthritis:

1 Control your weight
2 Enjoy gentle exercise
3 Get adequate sleep
4 Learn to relax
5 Have a good laugh

Control your weight

Extra pounds place excess wear and tear on joints and ligaments. Hundreds of diet plans exist to help you lose weight: ignore them all. The healthiest and most important step towards eliminating unnecessary fat from your body is to eat a balanced diet in moderation, and become more active. Using the *Eat to Beat Arthritis* Diet as your guide, choose foods that suit you best and enjoy them in small portions until your weight has reached an ideal level.

Serve yourself whenever possible (other people always give you more than you need), and only put on your plate what you intend to eat. Do not have second helpings. If you would usually take two tablespoons of peas, take only one. If you usually enjoy a full bowl of soup, ladle out half a bowl as your diet portion. For the good health of your heart and vascular system, cut the amount of butter and animal fat in

If you smoke, try to stop. The health evidence against smoking tobacco is overwhelming. Smokers dislike hearing people drone on about this, but the effects of smoke on your body are worth keeping in mind when you are committed to improving your health. As all those massively expensive anti-smoking campaigns tell us, the link between smoking and certain forms of cancer is obvious, but smoking causes other damage as well. There is evidence that the damaging levels of free radicals released in the body by cigarette smoke increases inflammation, and thus increases the level of pain associated with arthritis.

your diet to the smallest possible amounts, and use only half the oil you would usually use on salads and in cooking. Eat smaller portions and eat more slowly to enjoy the full flavour of your food. There are two exceptions to the rule on eating less. Among the foods you will enjoy on the *Eat to Beat Arthritis* Diet are liver and a nutritious Health Drink. Do not reduce your intake of either of these foods. (Gout sufferers must eliminate the liver, however. See page 67.)

If you are trying to lose weight, it is essential to add some extra exercise to your daily routine to burn off unwanted calories. Housework and walking to the shops are not enough.

Enjoy gentle exercise

Many of the causes of joint and muscle pain and discomfort should be eliminated or reduced by following the *Eat to Beat Arthritis* Diet. However, you also need to keep active to keep your body at its best, especially if you need to lose weight.

The choice of exercise activities is rich and varied. All you need to do is choose one and give it a try. If your first choice does not suit you, try another, and another, until you find one that you enjoy. Add at least three exercise sessions to your weekly routine. Include gentle stretching at both the start and conclusion of each session. No matter how old or unfit you are, visit the local gym and see if they offer anything that would interest you. Alternatively, contact local community and church groups to see if they offer activities that would get your blood pumping. You'll be surprised by the variety of activities available. For example, line dancing seems to be all the rage for every age these days, and some of the less strenuous martial arts both strengthen the body and calm the mind.

Remember, talk with your doctor before beginning any new exercise or sporting activity. He or she will probably applaud your decision to get out and get moving.

Good forms of exercise include walking, swimming and stretching. Gardening is also valuable exercise as it promotes joint health by stretching and placing gentle pressure on muscles surrounding joints in the arms, legs, hips and back.

Pain may be increased when you first start exercising, but you will soon 'work through' that as your stiff joints regain their flexibility. Exercise unlocks stiff joints and tissues. How many times have you heard someone say, 'I was so stiff this morning I thought I wouldn't be able to get out of bed; but once I got moving everything was fine.' You have probably had this same experience, and know that movement is a large part of keeping stiff limbs and muscles active.

To conquer the pain of arthritis, you should gently and repeatedly move the joints and tissues that hurt. By doing so, you strengthen the muscles that support the tissues, stimulate normal bone growth, and stimulate the circulation to the inflamed area. Remember, if you reduce your level of daily activity because you are afraid of the pain and discomfort that accompanies movement, you are going to lose more muscle strength and fail to stimulate normal bone growth.

Yoga and Pilates are two excellent exercise disciplines. Both stretch and strengthen muscles, but in their elementary forms neither one pushes or pulls muscles into extreme positions or activity. As relaxation is a principal goal in the practice of yoga, it has special value for arthritis sufferers. Yoga originated in India about three thousand years ago, and is based on physical control and relaxation. The practice has become increasingly popular over the past several decades, and many forms of movement and self-training have evolved. To learn more about yoga, visit your local library for books on the subject. Also, shop around to see what programmes are available in your area. Yoga is often offered in community and adult education centres.

Pilates is a form of exercise and body control developed by Joseph Pilates in the early 1900s. Born in Germany in 1880, Pilates was sickly and frail as a child, and as a result became obsessed by physical fitness. By the time the Great War broke out in Europe, Pilates was in England, teaching detectives self-defence. As a German, he was interned for the duration of the conflict. While in the camp he devised a regime of exercises for his fellow internees that maintained their health and fitness level while they were held in confinement. Not one of these people died during the influenza outbreak of 1918, and Pilates often claimed this was due to the exercise programme he developed. (There may be some truth in this, as we now know that exercise strengthens the immune system.)

After the war Joseph Pilates returned to Germany and began working with dancers and others who sought perfection in body form, flexibility and balance. When asked to begin work with the German army, Pilates refused and fled to America. On the boat he met a nursery teacher whom he later married. Together they established a fitness studio in New York, where dancers, athletes and members of top society soon became his clients. His devoted followers have included Martha Graham, Gregory Peck, Katharine Hepburn, Jodie Foster, Michael Crawford, Joan Collins and Sigourney Weaver. Tennis professional Pat Cash and world champion ice skating star Kristi Yamaguchi are among the athletes who have profited from Joseph Pilates' teaching. His methods are now taught around the world.

The Pilates method differs from other fitness programmes in the way the exercises are approached. Like yoga, it binds the activities of the mind with those of the body, making the mental perception of the body as important as physical movement. As in yoga, the three main elements of each exercise are relaxation, control and co-ordination. Pilates differs from yoga in one important way, however: the Girdle of Strength, that is the internal cage of muscles that supports and holds the body's internal organs in place, is tightened and used in every exercise practised. So too are the multifidous muscles, which stabilize the lumbar spine. By building power and flexibility into these often overlooked muscle groups, Pilates uniquely contributes to the physical fitness of sufferers of innumerable physical ailments and injuries.

For more about Pilates and how it can help you, browse in your local library and bookshop for more information. Also contact community and fitness centres to see what they have to offer in the way of basic courses.

Get adequate sleep

Insomnia affects the ability to concentrate and increases the awareness of pain and discomfort. If you have trouble sleeping, you are not alone. According to the Mayo Clinic in Rochester, Minnesota, more than 100 million people in the United States do not get a good night's sleep on a regular basis. Tired people have slower reaction times, are less productive and are less likely to interact with others in a positive manner. Like everyone else, arthritis sufferers should do all they can to maximize their chances of sleeping for eight hours a night. Here are some tips on what you can do to help you deal with this insidious problem.

First, however, what is insomnia? According to the Mayo Clinic, in the United States, these are some signs to watch out for:

- It takes longer than 30 minutes to fall asleep
- You wake several times during the night
- You wake up feeling muddled and tired
- You fall asleep during meetings and daytime events
- You are forgetful.

Dr Peter Hauri, Director of the Mayo Clinic Insomnia Program, suggests that answers to the following questions may help determine why you have sleep problems:

- Do you feel anxious when you are getting ready for bed?
- Do you argue with your spouse or partner in bed?

* Do you worry about the next day's tasks when you are trying to fall asleep?
* Do you keep checking the time on a bedside clock?
* Do you sleep better on holiday, or at a friend's house, than when you are in your own bed at home?
* Do you try to force yourself to go to sleep?

If you answered 'yes' to any of these questions you should take action.

Dr John W. Shepard Jr, M.D., Medical Director of the Mayo Clinic Sleep Disorders Center, has offered the following tips on how to get the full eight hours of sleep we all need each night. Remember, however, that what works for one person may not work for another. Try one or two of the following suggestions at a time until you find the combination that is right for you.

* Avoid caffeine and nicotine. Both are addictive stimulants that can interfere with sleep. (Remember that on the *Eat to Beat Arthritis Diet*, neither caffeine nor cigarettes are permitted.)
* Exercise, preferably in the afternoon.
* Watch what you eat and drink. Fatty and spicy foods may cause heartburn that disturbs sleep.
* Avoid drinking alcohol before going to bed; it may cause you to snore or get up during the night. (You should be avoiding it anyway while on the *Eat to Beat Arthritis Diet*.)
* If you must have a midnight snack, eat foods rich in the amino acid L-tryptophan, which triggers the release of serotonin in the brain. Good snacks include a glass of milk (warm or cold, as you prefer) or a tuna or turkey sandwich.
* Make sure the room is cool before going to bed, but have enough bedding to keep your body warm. Warm hands and feet encourage sleep.
* Avoid naps. Save your sleep for night-time.
* Enjoy stillness. Leave the radio and television off. If external noises disturb you use earplugs.
* Use your bed only for sleeping and sex. Watch television somewhere else.

- Set a sleep schedule. Try to go to bed and get up at the same time each day. Remember that a lazy Sunday morning in bed after a night out can mean a restless night ahead.
- Do not fret if you cannot go to sleep immediately. After a time, get up and do something else, like reading a good book. Then try again.

Learn to relax

Learn to unwind and let the world pass by. Use techniques like yoga and meditation to help release you from internal tension.

A hot bath or shower will relax you. Gently massage the area around inflamed joints. Try using herbal bath products that make you relax.

Many people who are disabled or slowed in their daily activities by pain become obsessive about what they *cannot* do. If this sounds familiar, then concentrate on what you *can* do, and do not be afraid to ask others for help to take care of the rest. It isn't easy, but it is necessary. If, for example, you are used to keeping your home and garden immaculate and can no longer do so, you need to admit that this is the case and take steps to reduce or spread the load. Decide which chores can be reduced in frequency, which can be turned over to someone else and which can simply be ignored. You may have ironed your bed linen – even your underwear – for many years but is it really necessary?

Have a good laugh

Laughter and a positive attitude are powerful medicines to be taken in large and frequent doses. When someone is in pain or discomfort they have a tendency to turn emotionally inwards. Before they know what has happened, the pain is worse. And as the pain gets worse, they withdraw into themselves. Laughter brings out the best in people. Let it lift you when those aching joints are getting you down.

To brighten your spirit:

* Enjoy films and videos that you know will make you laugh, even if you have seen them before. Read a book with a positive message. Better still, read a book of jokes or amusing short stories. I know a lovely elderly gentleman who reads Harry Potter to forget his gouty feet.
* Call a friend who makes you laugh. Avoid all talk of illness and pain; just enjoy a good chat.
* Write a letter to someone you love. Tell them about all the funny and happy things that you can remember happening during the past week.

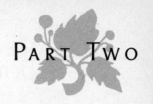

PART TWO

The Facts About Arthritis and Diet

CHAPTER 1

About arthritis

The aim in this part of the book is to get you started on the *Eat to Beat Arthritis* Diet. After basic information about arthritis in several of its more common forms you will read about food and diet, and how they affect inflammatory illnesses.

Coming from 'arthron', the Greek word for joint, *arthritis* literally means 'inflammation of the joint'. It may surprise you to know that about 200 different illnesses, all causing degeneration of joints and soft tissues, are classified as arthritis. Millions of people around the world suffer from some form of this illness, and in the United Kingdom one quarter of all visits to the doctor relate to its symptoms.

Although there are a surprising number of different types of arthritis, the great majority of people suffer from either *osteoarthritis* or *rheumatoid arthritis*. Both rheumatoid and osteoarthritis vary in their degree of severity, ranging from very mild discomfort to crippling. As you would expect, those with milder forms of these conditions will experience a greater degree of healing on this diet than those who have already suffered a major deterioration of joints. However, everyone should improve, and many will experience a return to normal activity.

Osteoarthritis is due to 'wear and tear' on joints, and most people beyond the age of 65 are affected to some degree. Athletes, or people involved in vocations that repeatedly use one or more joints – such as dancers and typists – may begin suffering from signs of arthritis at a relatively young age. Osteoarthritis may co-exist with other forms of arthritis, especially rheumatoid arthritis. It frequently occurs in the weight-bearing joints of the knees, hips and feet. Bony lumps, called 'nodes' sometimes form on the ends of finger bones, causing a gnarled, enlarged appearance. Stress, wear and tear can also cause slow deterioration of the discs between the spinal vertebrae, leading to pain and stiffness in the neck and back.

Heat and redness around an affected joint is common, and cold packs help dull the sensation of pain during the early part of an attack. Warm packs relax muscles surrounding joints, and are effective after acute pain has subsided. Remove warm packs after 10 minutes.

Rheumatoid arthritis is a chronic inflammatory disease involving the immune system. About three times as many women as men are affected. It is thought that some factor in the environment triggers an abnormal immune response in the joints. Many experts agree that specific foods may trigger inflammation. Unfortunately, not every case of rheumatoid arthritis responds to the same stimulus, and it is necessary to identify the specific food, or foods, that affect an individual.

Rheumatoid arthritis begins gradually with aching and stiffness. At first it may involve only one joint, but soon spreads to others, tending to affect the same joint on both sides of the body. Small lumps under the skin may appear around the elbows. Sufferers may get very tired, but experience a great deal of difficulty sleeping. A minority of sufferers will experience other symptoms, including skin rash and ulceration, enlargement of lymph nodes, and inflammation of tissues around the lungs and heart.

Bearing all this information in mind, just how does the *Eat to Beat Arthritis* Diet work? Its success relies on three objectives. The first is to eliminate from the diet all foods that trigger, or aggravate, abnormal inflammation in the joints and tissues. The second is to reduce the symptoms by supplying the body with nutrients known to strike at the stiffness, swelling and aching caused by inflammation. Many scientists believe that free radicals are a primary factor in causing inflammation, and foods used in the diet are rich sources of natural antioxidants that block inflammation. The third objective is to supply, through both food and dietary supplements, substances that help rebuild the internal components of joints destroyed by wear and tear.

Now that you know how the diet works, the following chapter will explain which foods are best for success.

Gout is a form of arthritis caused by a build-up of waste products in the blood. For more detailed information about it turn to page 233. For more detailed information on all forms of arthritis turn to pages 231–234.

CHAPTER 2

Food, supplements and medication

'People are more easily convinced of the power of magic, than convinced of the healing power of nutrition.'

The above statement – one I often use to open seminars – is, sadly, very true. Yet you *can* halt the pain of arthritis by changing the way you eat. In most cases, the difference will be so great it will change your life forever. All that is required for this transformation is the knowledge of which foods to avoid and which to enjoy, and a commitment to staying on the diet long enough to experience its benefits. Once you have experienced the improvement it brings about you will be very reluctant to return to your old ways. The path to success is not easy, however. You will be giving up foods and drinks that are part of most people's daily lives – for example, coffee, alcohol, bacon, bread and sugary sweets. These changes will be easier if you understand why they are necessary. Use this book as your guide, and you will soon find that you feel better, look better and no longer crave the foods that trigger the pain that once overshadowed your life.

Several years ago a group of women attending a community meeting about nutrition were asked for a show of hands as to how many agreed with the statement: *eliminating a single food from the diet can change a person's health.* Less than a third agreed. During the discussion that followed, some people were slightly amused by the question: after all, they ate a 'healthy' diet, how could that do them harm? When asked to describe a 'healthy diet', it was generally agreed that a healthy diet consisted of foods they 'had always eaten'. In fact, none of us eats 'what we have always eaten'. Differences in food production and processing – along with changing cultural influences – have subtly reshaped both the content and nutritional value of the food we eat. A healthy diet entails eating a high proportion of fresh fruits and vegetables, pulses, grains and nuts, and a modest amount of meat.

Many consumers are confused by all the dietary advice provided in the media these days. What should we listen to: old advice that we have followed for years; or new opinions still untested by time? Listen to both, and then ask yourself which makes good sense. If promises made for a wonder food sound too good to be true, they probably are. If someone tells you that a special diet will help control an illness, ask why and how it works. That is why you should take time to read all the information in this book, rather than just trying the recipes. You need to become familiar with your enemy in order to beat it.

Do eggs dangerously increase levels of blood cholesterol? The answer to this question is an example of how conflicting information about the health value of a food arises. Until the medical community became convinced that high levels of blood cholesterol were a significant risk factor in coronary artery disease, eggs were looked upon as a safe and healthy food, ideal for all the family – including infants and the infirm. Then came the theory that the cholesterol contained in foods, such as egg yolk, increases the level of blood cholesterol. As a result, people were advised to reduce their intake of eggs to as few as two per week. Recently, scientific research has established that the cholesterol contained in eggs has very little effect on blood cholesterol: saturated fats, such as those found in red meat, are the culprits. Eggs contain a far lower percentage of saturated fat than a portion of cheese of equal weight and, when enjoyed in moderation, they are an easy-to-eat food, high in the protein and vitamins our bodies need. Produced by free-range hens fed on grain and free of infection, eggs are a welcomed part of breakfast, lunch or dinner. You will see in Parts Three and Four that eggs are very much a part of the *Eat to Beat Arthritis* Diet.

Basic nutrition

Food is the essential link between your body and the rest of the living world. For optimum health, there is no substitute for a diet based on leafy vegetables, root vegetables, fruits, nuts, seeds, grains and various forms of meat. *Eat food in a form as close to its natural state as possible: fresh, raw or lightly cooked, unsalted and without artificial flavours, colours and preservatives.* That way, you will be giving your body the nutrients it requires.

Plants contain natural compounds that have healing properties. Ginger, for example, is not only a good source of B-vitamins, magnesium and zinc, but also contains a substance that helps control nausea. Chilli peppers contain a substance that fights pain. (More examples are found on page 38.) So to get the most from your diet, include a wide range of foods from plants, and vary what you eat.

A balanced diet contains a healthy combination of carbohydrates, proteins and fats. It may surprise you to know that international experts recommend a diet containing about 50 per cent carbohydrate, 30 per cent fat and 20 per cent protein. The healthiest carbohydrates come from grains, root vegetables and fruits. Sources of protein should be as low-fat as possible. Red meat (muscle) and full-fat milk products are high in saturated fats, which should be limited to no more than 10 per cent of the total calories consumed. Organ meats such as liver and kidney are relatively low in saturated fats, as are tofu and other plant-protein products.

It is widely believed that fats are bad for us, and that all fats should form a minimal part of a healthy diet. This is not true. Our bodies need fat, and deficiencies in certain fats lead to illness. Fats are a compact source of stored energy. They also aid the absorption of vitamins A, D and E from the gut, and form important parts of cell membranes, hormones and messenger molecules in the body. For good health, enjoy oils obtained from plants, and oily fish. These provide healing substances that people suffering from arthritis need to help fight pain. More is said about this when the omega-3 fatty acids, like those found in fish oil, are discussed. (See pages 236 and 251.)

If you are a vegetarian, ensure you eat at least one meal a day that *combines* grain and one or more pulses; for example, rice and beans. All the amino acids (protein building blocks) needed by the human body are found in plants, but not in the combination required by the human body. The amino acids we must obtain from our diet are called essential amino acids, and must be supplied in the same meal. More in-depth information can be found on page 247.

Vegetarians may not benefit from this diet as much as people who eat meat because they will not benefit from the healing properties of liver.

Foods that harm

Things we eat may cause harm in several ways:

- ❋ Some may contain a toxic substance that, eaten in excess, can create metabolic problems in your body.
- ❋ Some may trigger an allergic reaction.
- ❋ Some may cause food sensitivity.
- ❋ Some may aggravate inflammation.

Here are some examples:

Arthritis sufferers, and people concerned about the health of their bones, should be aware that rhubarb contains oxalic acid, which inhibits the body's ability to absorb calcium and iron from other foods. (The acid is concentrated in the leaves, which are poisonous and should never be eaten.) Rhubarb aggravates gout and rheumatoid arthritis, and may even cause an attack if eaten in excess. It may also increase the risk of kidney stones in some patients. If you cook rhubarb, do not use aluminium pans, as the acid juice dissolves aluminium from the surface, leaving it in the food for you to eat. Aluminium may be harmful to the body. Rhubarb is not the only plant containing oxalic acid. Smaller amounts are found in spinach, sorrel and chocolate.

Certain foods can trigger an allergic reaction – some people are allergic to nuts, for example. Seafood, especially lobster and prawns, may also cause problems.

This is a good opportunity to talk about the difference between an *allergic reaction* and *food sensitivity* (also known as *food intolerance*). These two conditions are frequently confused.

An *allergic reaction* is a serious matter that has immediate consequences. It is caused when the body's immune system has built up antibodies to one or more substances in a particular food. Symptoms include hives (urticaria), severe breathing difficulty, rash, swelling of the tongue and throat, and – in extreme cases – shock and death. Tingling of the lips and mouth after eating a particular food is a sign that an allergy to a particular food may be developing. If you experience such a response to a specific food, obviously it is prudent to avoid it.

Food sensitivity, or *intolerance*, is far less dramatic, but can cause serious symptoms that may vary from person to person. Migraine headaches, nausea, indigestion, eczema, stomach upset and hyperactivity have all been linked with food sensitivity. Symptoms do not appear with the speed seen in allergic reactions, and it is frequently difficult to identify the exact cause of the problem. In order to identify which food is causing the symptoms, an elimination diet is usually necessary.

For a few days the sufferer is placed on a diet based on foods known to cause little, if any, intolerance. This gives the body time to rid itself of substances that may be causing the problem. Following this rest period, other foods are introduced one at a time. Most will cause no recurrence of symptoms, and thereafter can be safely added to the diet. As more foods are introduced, almost inevitably one new item will cause symptoms to reappear. When this occurs, the culprit (or one of them) has been identified and the person on the exclusion diet will know to avoid that food in the future.

The *Eat to Beat Arthritis* Diet includes an elimination diet that should help you identify your sensitivity to foods that can trigger, or increase, the painful inflammation of arthritis.

Certain foods known to cause sensitivity are eliminated from the *Eat to Beat Arthritis* Diet. These are:

ALL PRODUCTS MADE WITH WHEAT AND OTHER GRAINS CONTAINING THE PROTEIN GLUTEN (RYE, BARLEY AND OATS)

More is said about this later (see page 48). For the moment, however, you need only be aware that gluten is often the cause of health problems ranging from migraine headaches to coeliac disease – a debilitating condition characterized by diarrhoea, bloating, and even anaemia. Coeliac disease can cause serious problems in some people, and even mimic the symptoms of certain forms of cancer.

Cutting out gluten will improve your general health and nutritional status. It will also help control the inflammation that causes much of the pain of arthritis.

ALL FOOD AND DRINK CONTAINING CAFFEINE

Some experts believe that caffeine increases the swelling and pain of inflammation. Many people find that removing this one source of trouble from their diet dramatically improves their life.

ALL PROCESSED FOODS, INCLUDING SALTED AND PRESERVED MEATS

Removing processed foods from your diet may seem daunting, but the rewards are great. You will be eliminating major sources of additives and unnatural chemicals from your body. You will be choosing not to eat foods that have been milled, stewed, or baked to the point that all the precious nutrients they once contained have been removed. And you will be leaving room in your diet for foods that are full of natural flavour and nutrition.

If you have gouty arthritis, the problem of diet becomes more complicated because liver and all other forms of offal should be avoided.

Foods that heal

How can something as basic as food heal? How can it be true that simply by changing the content of your dinner plate you can beat illness and heal damaged tissues?

Nothing in your body is static. Every moment of every day billions of cells are in constant change. They form, fill with molecules that conduct the chemical processes of life, and eventually die. It is said that over the course of seven years every molecule in the body is replaced. What we eat, and therefore supply to the body to reconstruct itself, determines its health and strength in the future.

When illness or injury damages the body, eating foods rich in the nutrients needed to replace and rebuild tissues promotes healing. When arthritis is present the nutrients most needed are protein; the B-vitamins, plus folic acid and biotin; vitamins C, E, B12, and D; the minerals selenium, manganese, iron, calcium and zinc; and certain specific fats known as omega-3 fatty acids.

The foods rich in these nutrients that form the basis of the *Eat to Beat Arthritis* Diet are:

* *Liver:* polyunsaturated fats, vitamin A, vitamin B2 (riboflavin), vitamin B3 (niacin), vitamin B5 (pantothenic acid), vitamin B12 (cobalamin), folic acid, biotin, selenium, copper
* *Kidney:* vitamin A, vitamin B2 (riboflavin), selenium, copper
* *Milk and dairy products:* calcium, zinc
* *Black treacle (molasses):* calcium, magnesium, zinc, iron
* *Brewers' yeast:* vitamin B1 (thiamin), vitamin B5 (pantothenic acid), vitamin B12 (cobalamin), folic acid, biotin, copper, magnesium, zinc
* *Oily fish:* omega-3 essential fatty acids, vitamin A,
* *Vegetable oils:* vitamin E, omega-3 essential fatty acids
* *Nuts and seeds:* vitamin E, manganese, magnesium, copper (omega-3 fatty acids are found in walnuts)
* *Fresh fruit and vegetables:* vitamin C, manganese

(More about healing foods can be found on pages 38 and 226.)

People with gout should enjoy celery and cherries several times a week. Both are thought to contain compounds that help the body eliminate uric acid. Celery also contains an anti-inflammatory substance.

Most of these nutrients play numerous roles in human metabolism. It is unnecessary to know all the details, but the following list identifies the specific role that makes them appropriate for arthritis sufferers:

- *Vitamin A* is needed for normal function of the immune system, and the control of inflammation.
- *B-vitamins* help maintain a healthy nervous system and fight depression.
- *Vitamin C* is needed to build collagen required for healthy tissues, including tendons and joints; it is also a strong antioxidant and fights damage by free radicals.
- *Folic acid* is needed for the normal absorption of other nutrients from the gut.
- *Vitamin D* plays a vital role in normal formation of bone.
- *Vitamin E* helps fight the oxidation of essential fatty acids in the body, thus reducing the symptoms of inflammation.
- *Selenium* is a strong antioxidant and helps protect against free-radical damage.
- *Magnesium* is an important component of bone.
- *Manganese* is vital for the normal formation of tissues in joints and bone.
- *Zinc* is essential for a normal immune system.
- *Copper* is needed for normal connective tissue and bones; it also helps protect against damage caused by free radicals and acts as an anti-inflammatory agent.
- *Omega-3 fatty acids* (as found in fish oil, hemp oil and walnuts) help control the inflammation, swelling and pain of arthritis.

The *Eat to Beat Arthritis* Diet recommends including frequent servings of offal such as liver, sweetbreads, heart and tripe. These are low-fat sources of protein that supply all the amino acids needed for healthy tissue. Sweetbreads contain useful amounts of important minerals, but not in quantities as large as those found in liver and kidney. Tripe and heart are good sources of low-fat protein, but contain smaller amounts of healing nutrients.

The BSE crisis in Europe forced the removal of many fine products from the market, and sweetbreads are among them. Very few stores now stock them, but a few organic meat producers have earned the right to sell these delicious morsels again. They are expensive, but when cooked correctly are delicious delicacies.

People with osteoarthritis will benefit significantly from eating foods rich in vitamin B12. The best source of these nutrients are the healthy bacteria in your own gut, but food sources are also available: liver and other animal proteins are a rich source, and play an important role in the *Eat to Beat Arthritis* Diet. If you are a vegetarian, vitamin B12 will be difficult for you to obtain from your diet. Plant sources include mushrooms and parsley. Certain fermented foods, such as tempeh and fermented black beans, contain a high bacterial count that insures they are a good source of vitamin B12.

PLANTS WITH HEALING POTENTIAL FOR ARTHRITIS SUFFERERS

- All fruits, except citrus, cranberries and plums.
- All green vegetables, except rhubarb and spinach.
- Broccoli, cauliflower, kale and cabbage are excellent sources of substances that fight cancer. (People with thyroid problems should limit their intake of these foods.)
- All root vegetables, with the exception of true potatoes. Sweet potatoes and yams are excellent for you, and full of texture and taste, as are Jerusalem artichokes and parsnips.
- Onions, garlic, leeks and shallots.
- Sprouted grains, beans and seeds. Mung beans and alfalfa are good. Sprouted brown rice is nice in a salad or stir-fries.
- Spices, especially turmeric and cinnamon.
- Seaweed, especially kelp, kombu and nori.
- All pulses (legumes), including aduki beans, black beans, soya beans, lentils, peas, chickpeas (garbanzo beans) and kidney beans. (People with gout should limit their intake of these foods.)
- Gluten-free grains: maize, millet, wild rice, brown rice, quinoa, buckwheat (kasha), amaranth. Avoid all products made with wheat, rye, barley or oats.

Dietary supplements and medications

The past ten years have seen a considerable increase in the number of medications available to treat all forms of arthritis. (The more frequently used of these are discussed on pages 234–235.) Although many people find these a primary avenue of relief from arthritis, they all carry some risk of side effects. The NSAIDS (non-steroidal anti-inflammatory drugs) can irritate the lining of the stomach and in some cases can cause ulcers when used over a long period. Commonly used NSAIDS include aspirin and ibuprofen. Treating arthritic symptoms by altering your dietary habits carries none of these risks.

The following dietary supplements have been shown to have special healing properties that counter the effects of both rheumatoid and osteoarthritis:

Vitamin E is one of the most powerful natural antioxidants identified to date. It works best when combined with vitamin C and the mineral selenium, both of which are well known for their antioxidant properties. Scientific studies have shown that people with rheumatoid arthritis have lower blood levels of antioxidants than others, and there is growing interest in what this means for the treatment of the disease. In a controlled study of osteoarthritis patients with knee and hip joint problems, 400mg of vitamin E was shown to be as effective in controlling symptoms as 50mg of Diclofenac, a medication classified as an NSAID. The effects of the NSAID were faster, but it produced more side effects than vitamin E. As pain relief over time was comparable, vitamin E was thought to be the treatment of choice.

Another study showed that rheumatoid arthritis patients treated with vitamin E had less pain and improved symptoms when treated over a three-month period. Vitamin E can be taken in large quantities with little risk of side effects.

Fish oil supplements are an important source of omega-3 essential fatty acids, and part of the *Eat to Beat Arthritis* Diet. You can read more about this subject on page 236. If you are a vegetarian, or cannot tolerate fish oil, try flaxseed oil instead. This is another rich source of omega-3 fatty acids, although they are in their original plant form, and have not been through the metabolic processes that produce the DHA and EPA fatty acids known to be deposited in the flesh of oily fish. These specific fatty acids are necessary for the body's production of small hormone-like molecules with strong anti-inflammatory properties, known as prostaglandins. Many people suffering from inflammatory illnesses experience dramatic effects when they supplement their diets with a fish or flaxseed oil supplement. For maximum benefit:

* Do not mix fish oil and other fatty acid supplements. Take omega-6 supplements (evening primrose oil or borage oil) at a different time of day.

* Make sure you take a vitamin E supplement, as this protects the omega-acids.
* Keep any opened bottles of supplements in the refrigerator or other cool place.

Note: there is a difference between *fish oil* and *fish liver oil*. Liver oils contain substantial quantities of vitamin A, which is stored in your liver and can be toxic if taken in large amounts. If you are setting out on this diet, it is recommended that you use *fish oil* supplements.

> Flaxseed oil is the richest known source of omega-3 fatty acids, and also contains substantial amounts of omega-6 fatty acids. It also contains plant chemicals known as *lignins*, which are plant estrogens that help control the body's estrogen level. Lignins are also believed to have other biological effects, including anti-viral and anti-bacterial activities.

Glucosamine and *chondroitin* are naturally occurring substances in the body that act as a building block in many tissues. Of the two, better curative effects have been demonstrated by glucosamine than by chondroitin, so it is suggested that this is the supplement of choice. Sometimes called the 'basement membrane builder', glucosamine is an essential substance in manufacturing and maintaining the ligaments, tendons, cartilage and synovial fluid found in joints. More detailed information on glucosamine and how it is thought to work can be found on page 237.

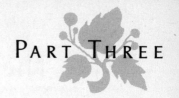

PART THREE

The Eat to Beat
Arthritis Diet

CHAPTER 1

The basics

What is the *Eat to Beat Arthritis* diet?

Since the 1930s, scientists have been aware of a possible link between rheumatoid arthritis and food allergies. Some scientists went so far as to suggest that symptoms of rheumatoid arthritis could be completely controlled by dietary changes.

Max Warmbrand, a naturopathic doctor who practised up until the mid-1970s, advocated a very low-fat diet in the treatment of both rheumatoid and osteoarthritis. In addition he told his patients to avoid eating all red meat, eggs, dairy foods, sugar, chemicals and processed foods. Six months were required before improvement was noticeable, he claimed. The diet seemed to work for a few people, but not others.

In 1979, Giraud W. Campbell wrote A *Doctor's Proven New Home Cure for Arthritis*, a book that helped millions of people break the bonds of this crippling disease. Using the information available at that time, he prescribed a strict regime that called for raw fruits and vegetables, hearty amounts of lightly cooked organ meats (liver, kidney, sweetbread, brain, heart and tripe), and daily doses of unpasteurized milk, nutrient-rich black treacle (molasses) and brewers' yeast. The diet began with a brief period of fasting, during which the body was freed of toxins from previous poor eating habits. He instructed his readers to shun all drinks containing caffeine, and cautioned against all processed foods – including canned and frozen items. If you followed this somewhat Spartan plan, you could end the pain of arthritis in seven days, he claimed.

The science of nutrition has changed greatly over the past several decades, and we know more about how and why you can control illness through diet. The *Eat to Beat Arthritis* Diet therefore builds on the Campbell diet, but also uses new information and a more modern approach to food and dietary supplements. At the same time, it recognizes some of the realities of modern life. For example, not all frozen foods are taboo: frozen peas, sweetcorn and spinach are very useful items in any kitchen. Soaking and cooking dried pulses such as chickpeas (garbanzo beans) takes hours; so canned ones, well rinsed to remove any salt and sugar, are allowed as an alternative.

This book also recognizes that more than seven days are needed to fully achieve benefits from recommended changes in food choices. Here, you will follow a gradual process that is tailored to your unique needs. The foundations of the *Eat To Beat Arthritis* Diet are:

* Finding the right balance of foods for your body.
* Knowing how to tell when a specific food is making the symptoms of arthritis worse.

The initial programme spans seven weeks. In the first week you keep a diary of your pain and stiffness and also record your intake of food and drink. You then learn to eliminate the specific foods that aggravate (or even cause) a flare-up of arthritis, and how to make this a diet you can use for life. You will also be encouraged to try new foods that you may have otherwise passed by.

While you remain on the *Eat to Beat Arthritis* Diet you will notice that you feel better. Depending on the severity of your condition you will find that pain will disappear, or diminish in severity. These are not the only exciting benefits you will enjoy from changing your eating habits. Selecting the right foods strengthens your body and enhances its metabolic activities. You will begin enjoying improved general health, stronger nails and hair and younger-looking skin. You will suffer from fewer colds and other infections. You may even find that you lose some of the excess weight that may be contributing to your joint pain and stiffness.

Rediscovering the way to eat

You are now ready to focus your attention on one of life's great plea-sures: food. What comes next will change your life forever. Previous sections of this book have covered three main topics:

- The causes and symptoms of several forms of arthritis.
- The links between good nutrition and healing.
- The role plant and other natural substances play in controlling pain and inflammation.

Armed with this knowledge, read the remainder of this book before you begin the diet. As you read, keep these principles in mind:

THERE ARE NO QUICK FIXES

If you follow this diet exactly, you will begin to feel better within days, but the full extent of healing will take longer. Diets promising remarkable cures often disappoint. If you really want to change the way you feel, and improve your health, you must be patient and give your body time to heal.

THIS IS A DIET FOR LIFE

A diet must be both practical and flexible, or you will find it boring and impossible. Once you have gone through a full seven-week cycle of the diet plan, you can occasionally bend the rules a little. In the chapter that follows, Marguerite discusses her flexible approach to the diet.

WHILE YOU ARE ON THIS DIET, ENJOY EATING

A partial list of the foods and ingredients you can incorporate into meals appears on pages 52–64. I call it a *partial* list because it cannot include every fruit, vegetable and fish from around the world. When you begin your new eating plan, take time to taste new vari-eties of fresh food. Have you tried the sweet, orange flesh of Sharon fruit? For a fantastic dessert, scoop out the flesh of chilled, ripe Sharon fruit and serve in small glass bowls. No sugar needed for this treat! On the more substantial side, have you enjoyed the delicate flavour of firm-textured steaks of escolar (mock sea bass), caught off the coast of South America? Or tasted barracuda fillets? If not, a treat or two awaits you.

The culinary arts are based on a rich palate of fruit, vegetables, meat, seafood, nuts, grains, seeds, herbs and spices. Combined in different ways by different cultures, these ingredients produce dishes with an endless variety of flavours and textures. The *Eat to Beat Arthritis* Diet actually sets very few restrictions on your enjoyment of this wonderful diversity.

THERE ARE CERTAIN FOODS AND DRINKS YOU MUST ABANDON

These are listed on pages 46–51. Don't let this put you off. Give your body a chance. Following the diet carefully for at least seven weeks should reduce the symptoms of arthritis and improve your general health, so it will be worth the sacrifice.

THERE ARE CERTAIN FOODS YOU MUST EAT

These are listed on page 35. Be faithful to these foods: they contain the healing nutrients your body needs. Include raw fruits and vegetables in your diet as often as possible.

THERE ARE CERTAIN DIETARY SUPPLEMENTS YOU MUST TAKE

Many of you will already be using supplements containing fish oil and vitamin E. The *Eat to Beat Arthritis* Diet also includes black treacle (molasses), brewers' yeast, and further suggests that you use supplements containing the mineral selenium (see page 241) and glucosamine, a naturally occurring substance that forms part of normal joint cartilage (see page 237).

DRINK WATER

This sounds simple enough, but you would be surprised how many people fail to drink enough water to fully flush waste products from their bodies. You need 1½–2 litres/2½–3 pints/1½–2 quarts, drunk in small amounts throughout the day. This can include fruit juice and milk, but no caffeine drinks. Filtered water and fresh tap water are recommended, or still bottled water (not carbonated).

Choose natural and organic foods

Avoid all foods contaminated with pesticides, additives, artificial sweeteners, preservatives, and anything else nature did not intend you to eat. Choose organic foods as far as your budget and their availability allow.

Enjoy your food raw or lightly cooked

Prolonged frying, boiling and baking destroy important nutrients and damage delicate molecules. Microwave cooking is quick and easy, and actually increases the availability of some nutrients in food. (There is no evidence that it 'denatures' food, as some people believe.)

If all this sounds a bit daunting, do not despair! You have a friend to talk you through it. In Part Four, along with the recipes she has developed for this book, Marguerite Patten gives you an insight into her own experiences on the diet, and answers practical questions about enjoying food and controlling pain.

The basic anti-arthritis diet: food and drink you must avoid

The first group to avoid is not only foods and drinks containing unnatural substances, but those that may have been contaminated by the environment in which they were grown or raised. The second group to avoid is food and drink known to cause food sensitivities, or to be potentially toxic to your body. The main offenders in both groups are detailed below.

Alcoholic beverages

Do your body a favour and eliminate this damaging substance from your diet. Here are a few facts to consider:

※ If you have ever suffered from a blinding hangover, you know that alcohol is toxic. Even in small amounts it can disrupt the natural biological functions of the liver, kidneys and heart. Large amounts can cause permanent damage.

* People who suffer from gout know that drinking alcohol can bring on an attack.
* The beneficial effects of certain medications – including antibiotics – are reduced by the consumption of alcohol.
* High alcohol intake increases the risk of certain cancers and heart disease.
* During pregnancy, alcohol can cause the growing foetus harm.
* Alcohol can increase depression and feelings of aggression. It is hard to stay on a diet – or any other health regime – when you lack self control or are in an irritable mood.

How can you have any kind of social life without enjoying a drink with your friends? Pubs and bars no longer look down on paying customers who ask for a glass of still mineral water on the rocks. In the right glass, it can look very drinkable indeed! Alternatively, try a glass of grape juice and pretend it is wine.

BEVERAGES CONTAINING CAFFEINE (COFFEE, COLA DRINKS AND TEA)

Coffee may be your favourite morning pick-me-up, but it plays nasty tricks on your body. It has been shown to increase inflammation, making an attack of arthritis worse. It can cause insomnia, robbing you of much-needed sleep. It can increase the rate at which minerals are lost from bone, escalating the possibility of osteoporosis. In large amounts it can cause heart palpitations and tremors of the hands. It also stimulates the secretion of stomach acid: if you suffer from heartburn it may be due to the coffee you drink. Coffee is addictive if taken frequently over a long period of time, so when you give it up don't be surprised if you experience some withdrawal symptoms for a day or two. Headaches are the most common problem.

All drinks containing caffeine create these problems to some degree. Remove all cola drinks, coffee and tea from your diet and you will soon find yourself free of some unpleasant symptoms you probably never associated with caffeine. Consider the following:

- Excessive amounts of caffeine increase the risk of osteoporosis in later life. This is particularly pertinent to women, who are far more prone to the condition than men.
- There is evidence that certain ways of brewing coffee increase the risk of heart disease.
- Caffeine is thought to increase blood cholesterol levels.
- Caffeine can make you jittery and tense, and alter your normal blood sugar levels.
- Migraine headaches can be triggered by caffeine.
- Caffeine acts as a mild diuretic. You are wrong if you think that all that coffee you drink helps satisfy your daily requirement for fluids – it does just the opposite. It draws precious water from your body and works the kidneys hard at the same time.

Many people find it harder to give up coffee than wine and spirits. Experts believe you can become 'hooked' on caffeine, and anyone who has gone off the brown stuff 'cold-turkey' will know how true this is. For this reason, we suggest you give up caffeinated drinks before you actually begin the diet.

A word about tea: it is off the *Eat to Beat Arthritis* Diet during the first two weeks, but then you can try a cup a day to see if your body will tolerate it. Tea contains certain powerful plant compounds with antioxidant and healing properties. A *single cup* of black or green tea each day may do you more good than harm.

ALL FOODS MADE FROM GRAINS CONTAINING GLUTEN
(WHEAT, RYE, BARLEY AND OATS)

For many people, simply eliminating gluten from their diet has changed their lives. It can do the same for you. Gluten is one of the most common causes of food allergies and sensitivities. It is a protein in plants that the human body does not use. However, because gluten gives food a nice texture, and a smooth, shiny appearance, it is used extensively by the food industry in the production of everything from baked products to stock cubes. Check everything you buy to make sure it does not contain gluten.

Sensitivities to gluten take many forms, including migraine, joint swelling and coeliac disease – characterized by dramatic diarrhoea and weight loss. Hair-like projections (the *villi*) absorb nutrients from food passing through the small intestine and transfers them into the bloodstream. Gluten can affect the *villi* by causing them to lie flat. This makes them less effective, thus restricting the amount of nutrients being absorbed the body. When this happens the person will become malnourished, no matter how much he or she may eat.

SUGAR

Although links have been suggested between high sugar intake and increased risks of diabetes, heart disease and certain types of cancer, none have been proven. What is certain, however, is that purified sugar gives you little more than empty calories that are easily converted to fat. Arthritis pain is made worse when unnecessary weight is placed on joints. So is sugar worth it?

Sugar also causes tooth decay and, by satisfying your hunger, discourages you from eating the complex carbohydrates (see page 249) needed to maintain a healthy blood sugar level.

Do not use artificial sweeteners. Natural substitutes for sugar are listed on page 52. Enjoy these instead, safe in the knowledge you are increasing your intake of beneficial nutrients.

CANNED AND PROCESSED FOODS

Just read the contents label on a can of soup or a packet of cake and you will see how many artificial ingredients are added to most processed food. Preservatives, artificial colours and artificial flavours are *not* part of the natural chemical composition of the human body. In addition, the nutrient content of many processed foods has been lowered during processing. So, with few exceptions, avoid canned and processed foods.

Many experts recommend the elimination of all canned and frozen foods. We do not agree. There are times when practicality and good sense must come into play. For example, made properly, houmous is a very good food. Few people make it for themselves because dried chickpeas (garbanzo beans) take forever to cook. Why not use canned ones, well washed and drained, to make your own? It's much better than being tempted by a store-bought variety or simply avoiding this nutritious dish.

Likewise, there are frozen foods that are at least as high in nutrients and as free from chemical residues as any you can buy in the fresh vegetable section of the supermarket. Best bets are frozen peas, corn (maize), spinach and beans. All these are usually frozen without the addition of any preservatives or other chemicals. (The very best, of course, come from your own organic garden, but few of us can enjoy such luxury.)

Smoked, pickled and cured foods

For thousands of years, humans have used these methods to preserve food during months of plenty in order to ward off starvation in times of want. They are unnecessary today because we have other ways of maintaining our food supply. However, because we like the taste of preserved foods – such as smoked salmon, pickled cucumber and bacon – preserved foods continue to play a large role in our diet. Unfortunately, these foods have drawbacks. All contain chemicals that are not naturally found in the human body, some of which carry potential danger. Both smoking and curing introduce chemicals into food that are known to be harmful and may be linked with certain forms of cancer.

Meat from factory-farmed animals

As the demand for food increases around the world, farmers are increasingly turning to the chemical industry for help. Hormones and antibiotics are used to increase growth rates, while chemicals are utilized to enhance animal health and cleanliness. As a result, food yields have increased dramatically over the past few decades. Careful health controls are in place to make sure that residues from these practices are held within 'safe' limits. But what are 'safe' limits?

One of the basic aims of this diet is to eliminate as many unnatural substances from the body as possible. So whenever possible, choose food that contains no – or at best low – levels of chemical residues. Press your local supermarkets to sell organic meat; increased demand will bring down the price.

NON-ORGANIC FRUITS AND VEGETABLES

Everything said about chemicals and meat is appropriate here. Carefully peel and wash all fresh fruits and vegetables not organically grown. To aid the release of dirt and chemical residue from grapes and berries place them in a glass bowl containing 3–4 tablespoons of vinegar to 1 litre (1 quart) of water; allow to stand for five minutes; rinse well and dry.

SEAFOOD CAUGHT IN INLAND STREAMS

Fish and shellfish are the best sources of protein you can have, and there are many varieties to choose from. But you must pick those that live in the deep waters of the seas and oceans.

The amount of industrial, agricultural and sewage pollution that finds its way into the waters of our once sparkling-clean streams and waterways means that pollution is a fact of life. Even in remote areas, environmentalists are finding increased levels of toxic substances. Some inshore waters are also affected – hardly surprising when effluent is pumped straight into them. Ask surfing enthusiasts about water pollution and you will hear gruesome details of contamination. All this, in turn, pollutes the fish we eat through the food they eat.

So choose fish from the sea or deep, clean Scottish lochs, and avoid adding your own body to the list of living organisms fouled by the waste in our water. Enjoy cod, bass, fresh tuna and game fish such as swordfish. If this sounds expensive, remember that your body requires no more than four or five ounces of protein a day. Smaller portions of fine fish makes sense.

The sad fact is that even our oceans are also slowly becoming polluted. Where will we go next for clean food?

The basic anti-arthritis diet:
food and drink you can enjoy

Those of you who suffer from gout should follow this advice, but avoid eating liver, kidney, spinach, sardines, shellfish, game, turkey, asparagus and rhubarb.

DRINKS

Fruit juice (see box below)
Fruit 'smoothies' (fruit, sometimes combined with milk or yoghurt, put through a blender)
Milk (the base of your daily Health Drink, see page 71)
Tea (for the first two weeks drink only herbal tea. After that one cup of black or green tea a day is allowed)
Water (cool, freshly filtered water, tap water or still bottled water)

Fruit juice is a delicious part of this diet. Buy a juicer and make your own, or use concentrates prepared with no preservatives. Ask your health-food store to stock brands made from organically grown fruit. Recent years have seen some excellent products come on to the market.

SWEETENERS

Black treacle (molasses)*
Honey (organic)
Cactus syrup
Maple syrup
Date syrup (yummy!)
*Puréed fruit*** (apricot purée makes a wonderful sauce, or can be served with yoghurt as a tasty dessert)
Concentrated fruit juices (organic and free of preservatives)

*Black treacle (molasses) is an important ingredient in the *Eat to Beat Arthritis* Diet, as it is a healthy source of calcium, magnesium and phosphate, all of which are needed for healthy bones. It is also rich in iron, copper and zinc, and contains traces of several B-vitamins.

**Puréed *dried* fruits are an excellent source of nutrients. Dried apricots are especially good because they contain: beta-carotene (a powerful antioxidant and the substance your body needs to make vitamin A); fibre needed for a healthy digestive system; B-vitamins used during metabolism and functioning of the nervous system. (Apricots are also an excellent source of folic acid, a member of the B-complex, which is vital for the production of blood cells and the normal development of the foetal nervous system. Recent evidence suggests that it is also needed for a healthy heart.)

BAKED GOODS AND PASTA

You can enjoy all baked goods and pasta made with organic, *gluten-free* flour. There are some excellent products on the market, but also try making your own. Do not simply substitute gluten-free flour for that specified in standard recipes; use recipes tried and tested on the product. And, if you plan to use a bread machine, make certain your recipe and ingredients specify that they are appropriate for that purpose.

OILS AND FATS

*Butter**

Canola (rapeseed) *oil**

*Corn oil**

Groundnut (peanut) *oil* (unless there is evidence of an allergy)

*Olive oil**

Safflower oil

*Soya oil**

*Sunflower oil**

Sesame seed oil

Walnut oil

**Butter* is an enjoyable source of flavour in food. Used in small amounts it can make a world of difference. Remember, however, that it is a saturated fat, which should make up no more than 10 per cent of your total caloric intake. Also, it contains traces of milk protein. Some people sensitive to cows' milk may find it causes phlegm or other symptoms. Clarified butter can be a substitute.

**Olive oil* is an excellent ingredient for dressing salads and vegetables, and for cooking. It is a rich source of the fat we need in greatest quantity:

oleic acid, a monounsaturated fat. Olive oil is low in saturated fats, and contains antioxidants and plant compounds that have been shown to have healing properties. Choose a good-quality olive oil, even though the price may seem high. There are several grades of olive oil on the market: extra-virgin is the most expensive. It is worth the money, however, because it has been subjected to the least mechanical processing. Dr. Robert Owen and colleagues at the Division of Toxicology and Cancer Research Factors, German Cancer Research Centre, Heidelberg, have recently stated that the unique blend of compounds in olive oil giving it health-promoting properties are lost during processing.

Sunflower oil, safflower oil, corn oil, canola (rapeseed) oil and *soya oil* are all sources of essential fatty acids needed for good health. Do not overheat them as their delicate molecular structure is damaged by high temperatures. Keep all oils in a cool dark place, and discard if they begin to have a strange fishy smell; this means they are rancid.

Fruits

Avoid canned fruits unless there is no alternative, because canning removes nutrients found in fresh products. Rinse well before using to remove any additives and contaminates from cans. Even then, limit your intake. For example, canned pineapple is permitted, but infrequently. Frozen fruit is fine as long as it does not contain added sugar or preservatives.

Apples – in all their delicious varieties
Apricots – loaded with vitamins and minerals. Fresh are best, but you can also enjoy dried ones provided they are prepared with no preservative
Avocados – include this delicious fruit in your anti-arthritis diet whenever possible
Bananas – a great source of energy and nutrients
Berries – strawberries, raspberries, loganberries, blueberries, cranberries, blackberries, currants (red and black), gooseberries and anything

else that falls into this category. Many berries contain phytochemicals with natural antiviral and anti-bacterial properties, so they give your body an extra edge when fighting off infection

Cherries – another red fruit loaded with natural healing substances for your body

Currants

Figs – great flavour and highly nutritious. Fresh are best

Grapes – red or black are best, as they contain more natural antioxidants, but white ones will do

Guava

Kiwi fruit

Mangoes – sweet, smooth, and an excellent source of vitamins

Melons – a versatile low-calorie food that can be used in salads, main courses, desserts and even soups!

Papaya (*paw-paw*)

Peaches – excellent source of flavour and nutrients. Fresh are best

Pears – fresh are best

Plums

Prunes

Raisins

Sultanas

> Note: this list does not include citrus fruit. This is because many people are surprised to find that their arthritis symptoms greatly improve when they eliminate oranges, lemons, limes and grapefruit from their diet. You will read more about this later. For now, just remember that citrus fruit is not part of the Basic Anti-arthritis Diet.

VEGETABLES

Beetroot (*beet*)

Broad beans (*fava beans*)

Broccoli

Brussels sprouts

Cabbage – all forms
Cardoon
Carrot
Cassava
Cauliflower
Celery – gout sufferers should include celery in their diet at least three times a week
Chard
Chicory
Chives
Courgettes (zucchini)
Cress
Cucumbers
Endive
Fennel
Garden peas
Garlic
Globe artichoke
Green beans
Horseradish
Jerusalem artichokes
Kale
Kohlrabi
Leeks
Lemongrass
Lettuce – all types
Lima beans
Lotus root
Mangetout (snow peas)
Marrow
Mushrooms
Okra
Olives
Onions
Pak choi
Plantain

Parsley – parsley is considered a vegetable here because it is so rich in nutrients
Parsnips
Peas, garden
Pumpkin
Radishes
Shallots
Sea vegetables – including *agar-agar, carragheen, dulse, kelp, nori (laver)* and *wakame*
Sorrel
Spinach
Squash – summer and winter
Spring onions (scallions, green onions)
Swede (rutabaga)
Sweetcorn (corn on the cob)
Sweet potato
Swiss chard
Turnips
Yam (yellow and cush-cush)
Water chestnuts
Watercress

> You will notice that several very popular vegetables are missing: tomatoes, potatoes, peppers and aubergines (eggplants). This is because they are all members of the nightshade family of plants, and cause food sensitivities in some people. Leave these off the menu during the first two weeks of the diet. You may be able to reintroduce them later if you prove not to be sensitive to them.

PULSES (LEGUMES)

These foods can be enjoyed fresh, canned, frozen or dried. Canned are often preferable as they are easy to use and will have been well cooked (this applies especially to kidney beans as they contain toxins which must be removed by rapid boiling). However, you must drain and rinse them well. People with gout should avoid pulses as they contain purines.

Beans of all kinds:
aduki, borlotti (pinto), broad (fava), brown, butter, cannellini, flageolet, ful medames, haricot (navy), red and *black kidney*
Blackeyed peas
Chickpeas (garbanzo beans)
Lentils – red, green and brown
Mung beans
Peas, whole and split
Soya beans (all foods made of soya are rich in plant chemicals that help protect the body against cancer and heart disease)

GRAINS
Amaranth and *Quinoa* – two grains from South America with a high protein content
Buckwheat – not a type of wheat, but seeds from a plant in the rhubarb family
Corn (maize)
Millet – an excellent source of vegetable protein
Rice – brown is preferable to white as it contains more nutrients
Wild rice – not a true rice, but seeds from a North American grass

Substitutes for wheat flour include:
Arrowroot (ground)
Buckwheat flour
Cornflour (cornstarch)
Corn meal (maize meal)
Gram flour – ground *chickpeas (garbanzo beans)*
Potato flour – check for sensitivity before using this
Rice flour
Soya flour

> Grains: gluten is a major cause of food sensitivity. Wheat, rye, barley and oats should be completely avoided. However, as grains are the main source of B-vitamins and minerals, forming an important part of a balanced diet, you need to find gluten-free alternatives.

NUTS AND SEEDS
Nuts
Almonds
Brazil nuts
Pine (pignolia) nuts
Walnuts

Seeds
Alfalfa
Fennel
Linseed
Mustard
Pumpkin seeds
Sesame seeds
Sunflower seeds

HERBS AND SPICES
You can eat as many herbs and spices as you like. There are none that will harm you when eaten in moderate quantities, and many contain healing and nutritious substances that are a welcome part of a healthy diet.

EGGS AND DAIRY FOODS
Forget the terrible things you have read about eggs in the past. Research has shown they make little difference to blood cholesterol, but are an excellent source of nutrition. Just make sure they are fresh and from a source you trust. Organic eggs are best; failing these buy ones from free-range grain-fed chickens. Vary your menu by trying quail and duck eggs in addition to hen's eggs.

Some people find eggs constipating, but this is usually due to lack of sufficient high-fibre foods. If you are eating the amount of fruit and vegetables specified in the diet you should have no problems.

Dairy foods are excellent sources of calcium and protein, which are both needed for healthy bones. Cheeses and yoghurt of all kinds are good for you, but remember:

- Yoghurt should be unsweetened – add honey, date syrup or fruit if necessary.
- Avoid processed cheeses such as spreads, Gruyère triangles and low-fat types. Keep to natural cheeses, such as Cheddar, feta, Edam and full-fat cottage cheese.
- Dairy products are rich in saturated fat, and therefore should not be the major source of protein in your diet.
- When Dr Giraud Campbell wrote his diet, in the late 1970s, food contamination was a far less significant problem than it is today. He recommended drinking a glass of unpasteurized milk each day: we do not. Drink full-fat pasteurized milk from a reliable source. Some people are allergic to cows' milk – excessive phlegm and coughing are common symptoms. If you think you may be susceptible, eliminate cows' milk from your diet for two days, substituting soya milk, or pasteurized goats' or ewes' milk.

Fish and Shellfish
All deep-water fish, including:

Abalone
Anchovy
Barracuda (becune, sea pike)
Bass
Bluefish
Bonito
Bream
Brill (britt, kite, pearl)
Cockles (arkshell)
Cod

Coley (coalfish, pollock, saithe)
Conger eel
Clams
Crabs
Croaker (black drum, queenfish, sea drum, weakfish)
Cuttlefish
Dogfish (flake, huss, rigg, tope)
Dolphinfish (dorade, dorado, lampuka, mahi-mahi) – these are *not* dolphins
Flying fish
Grey mullet
Grouper
Gurnard
Haddock
Hake
Halibut
Herring
John Dory (tila pia)
Langoustine (Dublin bay prawns)
Lemon sole (lemon fish, lemon dab)
Lobster
Monkfish (anglerfish)
Mussels
Octopus
Oysters
Pompano
Prawns
Redfish (berghuilt, Norway haddock, ocean perch, red perch, rose fish)
Red mullet
Red snapper
Salmon (wild is preferable, but is very expensive and may not be readily available. Farmed salmon is acceptable so long as it comes from deep Scottish lochs)
Scabbard (espada, sabre fish)
Scallops
Sea bream (porgy, scup)

Shark
Shrimp
Skate
Sole
Squid (calamar)
Swordfish
Tuna – not canned
Turbot
Whiting

- Enjoy the roe from any of the above. If the budget allows, salmon roe and caviar are excellent sources of nutrients. Unfortunately, people with gout should avoid all fish roe (eggs) because they are high in purines.
- Avoid smoked or commercially salted fish.
- Gout sufferers should ask their doctors if it is okay for them to eat shellfish and anchovy.

Offal (organ meat, variety meat)

Offal is a general term used to describe the internal organs of an animal, and includes liver, kidney, heart, brain, tripe and sweetbreads (the pancreas and thymus gland). These form an important part of this diet. Liver is the most nutritious offal, and is an excellent source of many important nutrients needed to heal tissues and control the symptoms of arthritis. Since the BSE outbreak in Europe, brain is no longer recommended.

Unfortunately, people with gout should avoid eating all types of offal because of its high purine content.

Liver

This highly nutritious meat is the most important food in the *Eat to Beat Arthritis* Diet. Try including it in your menu at least three times a week. Liver is rich in vitamin A, pyridoxine (vitamin B6), cobalamin (vitamin B12), riboflavin (vitamin B2), niacin, folate and biotin; also the minerals iron, selenium, zinc, molybdenum and copper. It is also a good source of pantothenic acid (vitamin B5), calciferol (vitamin D), and co-enzyme Q10.

Do not overcook liver, as some of the more delicate nutrients will be lost. It is also much nicer to eat when it has just turned colour and is still soft – not grey and hard.

KIDNEYS
Kidneys are less rich in nutrients than liver, but still rank among the best. Kidney is a rich source of riboflavin, biotin, vitamin B2, vitamin B12, iron and niacin. It also contains useful amounts of the minerals zinc, selenium and molybdenum. It also contains useful amounts of vitamin A.

HEARTS
These are a rich source of choline and inositol. These substances help prevent fatty degeneration of the liver, and choline is part of the chemical complex involved in the transmission of nerve impulses.

SWEETBREADS
This delicious food is the thymus gland and pancreas taken from calves, lambs and pigs. Considered by many to be a great delicacy, they may be both hard to find and expensive. Sweetbreads are an excellent source of zinc, several of the B-vitamins, and minerals.

TRIPE
Tripe is the muscular part of the stomach, and an excellent source of almost fat-free protein. However, it has few of the nutrients for which liver and kidneys are prized. If you do not like it, skip it.

GAME ANIMALS
If cooked well, wild game – rabbit, hare, venison and wild boar – are delicious alternatives to the usual forms of meat.

FARMED MEAT
All cuts of beef, lamb, pork, veal, kid and goat are acceptable – though you should always try to buy organic meat. If this is not possible, purchase from sources where you know that only the minimum amount

of antibiotics, hormones and other foreign substances are used in raising the animals and preparing them for market.

Remember, however, that red meat is a rich source of saturated fat, which should be kept to a minimum on a healthy diet.

Avoid all forms of cured, processed and salted meats, including bacon, ham, sausages and salami. Vegetarians should turn to pages 32 and 247, where they will find advice on obtaining the essential amino acids that are normally provided in the diet through eating meat.

POULTRY AND GAME BIRDS
Domestic – organic
Wild game birds are often preferable to poultry, unless the latter is organically produced.

Chicken (avoid capons)
Duck
Goose
Turkey (because of its high level of purines, this meat should be avoided by people with gout)

Game birds
Guinea fowl
Grouse
Quail
Partridge
Pheasant
Pigeon
Snipe
Squab
Wild duck
Woodcock

CHAPTER 2

The seven-week diet plan

Read this chapter carefully before you begin. You may also find it useful to read Part Four, in which Marguerite Patten recounts her experience on the diet, and gives tips on how to succeed.

Seven weeks may seem like a long time, but it is a worthwhile investment in your health.

The aims of the diet plan are:

- To become more aware of what you eat, and identify the pattern of your pain and discomfort (Week Zero).
- To introduce high-nutrient foods and food supplements that will reduce inflammation and encourage healing in joints and surrounding tissues (Week One).
- To give your body an opportunity to rid itself of the effects of foods to which you are sensitive (Weeks One and Two).
- To eliminate from your diet any foods that may increase joint inflammation (Weeks One to Seven).

Not everyone responds at the same rate. Some people take longer to notice an improvement than others. Full benefits from this plan depend on which type of arthritis you have, and your body's sensitivity to specific foods. Soon after you begin this diet plan, you should feel better and have less pain. It may be tempting to rest on one's laurels then, and not continue with the full seven-week plan. Please give your body time to heal and adjust to this new plan of foods and supplements, and stay with the diet for the full seven weeks to receive its full benefit.

Week zero

Unlike most diets, where you just plunge right in, this one involves taking time to prepare yourself for the changes you are about to undertake. Knowing yourself – your feelings and your body – is the keystone to improving your health.

Too many of us begin diets with good intentions and high expectations, but lack a realistic view of what lies ahead. It is human nature to want a quick fix when in pain or ill. We expect changes in ourselves to take place overnight. When that does not happen, we get discouraged. We may stick to a diet for weeks, or even months, but slowly old habits creep back. However, if you can actually see improvements, by recording your body's response to your new eating habits, you are more likely to stay the course.

> If you smoke, seriously consider ridding yourself of this addiction. Along with being a cause of cancer and a predisposing factor in heart disease, it speeds up the ageing process and damages tissues – including those found in joints. Give it up!

During this week of preparation there are two aims:

* To better understand your pain and discomfort, and your dietary habits, by using a self-assessment diary.
* To eliminate all caffeine and caffeine-like substances from your body.

Let us deal with this second aim first. 'Why', you may ask, 'begin eliminating anything from my diet before Week One?' The answer is simple: caffeine increases the pain of inflammation; it is also mildly addictive. Too much caffeine can cause jittery feelings, and add to aggressive behaviour and even tremors.

People who drink four or five cups of coffee – or fewer very strong cups – each day find they experience headaches, tiredness and irritability when they stop. These symptoms can be mild, or surprisingly uncomfortable. They may appear a few hours after you stop drinking caffeine – or not at all. As you *must* eliminate caffeine from your diet, it is best to deal with this beast before tackling other foods and drinks that may be causing you trouble. You will be delighted by the effect this has on your body. Joint pain frequently dramatically improves. A feeling of calm, and being in control, often sets in. You will sleep better, look better and feel better. What better reasons could there be for giving up something your body does not need, and that ultimately increases your pain?

The other aim for Week Zero, better understanding of your pain and discomfort, and your dietary habits, is achieved by using a self-assessment diary. Draw out a basic format and fill it in meticulously – see sample forms on the following pages.

WARNING!

If you know you have gout, *do not* eat liver, kidney, heart, sweetbreads or tripe. Offal is high in purines, which should be avoided. Poultry and pulses are also high in purines. For protein in your diet, substitute game, pork, lamb, deep-water fish and soya products such as tofu. Add high-quality multivitamin and multimineral supplements to your diet regime to replace the natural nutrients you would otherwise obtain from liver and other organ meats. Make certain the mineral supplement contains selenium.

Sample Self-Assessment Form

Week zero, day 3 Time	Week zero Meals, snacks and drinks	Pain and discomfort location, severity (1–5)
7 A.M.–10 A.M.		
10 A.M.–1 P.M.		
1 P.M.–5 P.M.		
5 P.M.–12 Midnight		
Midnight–7 A.M.		

Sample Completed Self-Assessment Form

WEEK ZERO, DAY 3 TIME	WEEK ZERO MEALS, SNACKS AND DRINKS	PAIN AND DISCOMFORT LOCATION, SEVERITY (1–5)
7 A.M.–10 A.M.	Wheat toast with butter 2 fried eggs with bacon Coffee, milk and sugar Orange juice – 8fl oz (1 cup)	Stiff knee and back on rising (3) Knee worse late morning (4)
10 A.M.–1 P.M.	Coffee and biscuit – 11.00 Note: coffee should have been eliminated from the diet by this time	Knee red and painful after walking dog (5)
1 P.M.–5 P.M.	Lunch – tuna and tomato sandwich with cola drink; Chocolate bar; Herbal tea with milk and sugar; Scone with butter and jam	Hip hurt after lunch (3) Lay down to rest
5 P.M.–12 MIDNIGHT	Dinner – roast chicken potato and gravy, peas and carrots, Herbal tea and cake for dessert	Hip very sore (5) Took hot shower to relax it
MIDNIGHT–7 A.M.	Glass of water before bedtime	Could not sleep Pain in hip and knee (3)

Week One – the elimination diet

To begin this all-important part of the plan, organize your self-assessment diary for the week. Make a commitment to yourself that you will record details of how you feel and what you eat each day. These notes form the picture that will show how you are progressing.

REMEMBER:

* Eliminate all wheat, rye and barley from your diet. For now, do not eat oats in any form.
* Say goodbye to caffeinated drinks: coffee, tea, cola and chocolate.
* Say goodbye to all alcoholic beverages.
* Eat food raw when possible. Otherwise cook it lightly to maintain maximum nutrients.
* Drink 4–5 glasses of fresh water each day.
* If you are sensitive to cows' milk, drink goats', ewes' or soya milk instead.
* Eliminate all processed foods from your diet.
* Eliminate all sugar and artificial sweeteners from your food.
* For now, *do not* eat citrus fruit, asparagus, all red meat, tomatoes, aubergine (eggplant), all forms of peppers, and 'true' potatoes (sweet potatoes and yams are permitted).

Until you reach Weeks Three to Six, avoid eating all foods containing high levels of oxalic acid: rhubarb, cranberry, plum, chard, beet greens and spinach.

DAY ONE

A day of fasting is a good way to begin an elimination diet. This should be a time to pamper yourself – so stay warm, rest, and sip cool, fresh water. If you get terribly light headed, sip a glass of fruit juice. *Remember:* citrus fruit and tomatoes are off your diet for now, so choose peach, mango, grape or cherry juice. This is the only day you can skip the Health Drink.

DAY TWO

Today you can eat three light meals all based on raw fruit and vegetables. One of these should contain some liver. Sautéed liver and onions are always a treat.

Beginning on Day 2, take capsules containing the equivalent of 1 gram of fish oil, or take 2 tablespoons of cod liver oil each day. Fish oil is the better choice. All fish liver oils are rich in vitamins A and D, which accumulate in the liver and can be toxic in large quantities. Fish oil does not carry this risk. If you take these supplements with food they are less likely to 'repeat' on you. *If you have diabetes, or are on any medication that thins the blood, please ask your doctor before adding this supplement to your daily diet.*

HEALTH DRINK

On Day 2 add your daily Health Drink. Mix 225ml/8fl oz/1 cup of whole, pasteurized milk with 1 tablespoon of dried brewers' yeast and 1 tablespoon of black treacle (molasses). You may find that mixing these ingredients in a blender with a small banana makes a more palatable drink. Do not use bakers' yeast; use only brewers' yeast, and avoid unpasteurized milk.

DAY THREE

The same as day two but add seafood from deep-water sources. It is also suggested that on Day 3 you add 400 i.u. of vitamin E to your diet. The anti-ageing benefits of this vitamin not only support healthy joints, but also protect the heart.

DAYS FOUR, FIVE, SIX AND SEVEN

The same as the above. Each day enjoy one meal containing seafood and one based on an organ meat.

At the end of Week One, find a comfortable chair, put your feet up, and have a long look at your self-assessment diary. Have you noticed any changes in the level of discomfort or pain you are experiencing? If you suffer from joint stiffness, is it about the same as at the beginning of Week Zero? Does it occur at the same times during the day, or has this changed? Make a few notes to summarize any changes, and add a sentence or two about how you feel about the diet.

Constipation: for good health you should avoid constipation and straining when having a bowel movement. Some other diet books, including that written by Giraud Campbell, recommend colon cleansing, or enemas; we do not. The only function of the colon is to absorb water and salts from the digestive residue carried through the system by the gut. Bacteria and waste materials accumulated during digestion are naturally eliminated by the muscular contractions of a healthy colon. Many medical doctors treating digestive illnesses do not recommend colon cleansing because it disrupts the functions of the lower bowel.

To avoid constipation and straining, drink 8–10 glasses of water every day and follow the *Eat to Beat Arthritis* Diet. The wide selection of fresh fruits and vegetables you enjoy will supply at least the 20–30 grams of natural fibre you need each day for a healthy digestive system.

Week Two – resting your body

Continue the diet you followed on days 4, 5, 6 and 7 of Week One.

Do not forget the Health Drink of milk, black treacle (molasses) and brewers' yeast.

Remember to take the recommended amounts of fish oil and vitamin E.

If you have experienced little or no improvement thus far, and are drinking cows' milk and/or eating cheese made from cows' milk, eliminate these products from your diet. Substitute goats', ewes' or soya milk.

At the end of Week Two, reassess your pain and stiffness. Write down a summary of your experience, and also record how you are feeling on the diet. Have you lost a bit of unwanted weight? How is your skin? Some people find that by this time their skin has a fresher look and they have fewer blemishes.

SOME THINGS ARE NOT FOREVER –
ELIMINATING FOOD SENSITIVITIES AND ALLERGIES

By eliminating the most common causes of food sensitivity during the first two weeks of the *Eat to Beat Arthritis Diet,* your body has been refreshed. Unfortunately, some of your favourite foods may be missing from your table during this process. Cooking without any potatoes, tomatoes or peppers can be difficult, but the results will make the effort worthwhile. Delicious recipes and tips to help get you through this phase of the diet are provided in Part Four. Do not despair. You need not give up all these foods forever. From the beginning of Week Three you can begin testing various foods to see how your body responds.

Weeks Three to Seven – learning to expand your food vocabulary

Now that your body has been resting on an allergen-free diet for two weeks you have reached the time when you can come to grips with how it reacts to specific foods known to cause problems. Because it takes three days to test each food, or food group, this takes some time, but the results are well worth it. Remember to have your Health Drink each day.

The process of testing your sensitivity to a food is simple:

* Add a new food, or group of foods, to your diet by using it in some wonderful dish you enjoy. Have it for lunch or dinner. Keep notes in your self-assessment diary of any twinges you may have.
* The following day, have the same food again – perhaps prepared in another way. Are there any new twinges of discomfort? Or, is your stiffness worse, or about the same?

❄ Go back to the Basic Arthritis Diet for a day, and see how you feel. If your arthritis has shown no signs of getting worse at the end of the third day you can be fairly certain that the food you have reintroduced is not making your arthritis worse. Add it to the list of foods you can eat, and enjoy!

❄ Go on to the next food, or food group, listed below, and use the same three-day test to see how your body responds. Continue until you have covered the entire list.

Remember that *allergies* and *sensitivities* are not the same. If you begin to feel a tingling feeling around your mouth soon after eating a specific food – such as lobster – you are probably allergic to it. Symptoms may get worse, and you may experience swelling in your mouth, or shortness of breath. If this occurs, seek medical help at once. In their most extreme form, food allergies can lead to anaphylactic shock and death. Other allergy symptoms are eczema, asthma, and hives (urticaria). If any food gives you a hint of these symptoms *eliminate it from your diet at once and for good*.

It is important that you test foods in the order listed below

1 All dairy food made from cows' milk, known as bovine products. Cows' milk is not well tolerated by many people because they are unable to digest the protein in milk and cream. Physical symptoms include inflamed and swollen joints, and phlegm. If you develop a cough a few hours after breakfast, do not be surprised. What may appear to be an on-coming cold could be a reaction to the milk you poured on your morning cereal.

If you find you experience symptoms at this stage, check to see if you can tolerate cheese and yoghurt. Eliminate milk and cream from your diet for 48 hours, and then try only yoghurt and cheese. The protein in these products has been altered by natural processes, and is more easily digested.

2 All citrus fruits: oranges, tangerines, satsumas, clementines, lemons, limes, grapefruit and kumquats. (This includes your morning glass of orange juice! Some people find that the simple elimination of orange juice dramatically reduces joint pain.)

3 Foods high in oxalic acid: spinach, rhubarb, cranberries, plums, chard and beet greens. (If you have gout, don't even test yourself for these foods: eliminate them from your diet now and forever.)

4 Asparagus. (Asparagus is high in purines and should be avoided by those with gout.)

5 Cheese made from buffalo milk (authentic mozzarella). Sensitivity to products made from cows' milk (bovine milk) may mean you are also allergic to buffalo milk. But if you find you are not affected, then this is a great food to include in Mediterranean dishes.

6 Nuts, with the exception of almonds, walnuts and pine (pignolia) nuts, which are part of the Basic Anti-arthritis Diet.

7 Nightshade vegetables: tomatoes, aubergine (eggplant), peppers and 'true' potatoes. These should be the last test foods in your arthritis diet plan. The substances they contain, which are mildly toxic in some people, take a long time to work their way through the body.

If pain reoccurs go back to Week One and begin again.

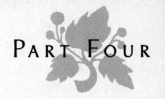

PART FOUR

The Recipes

Contents

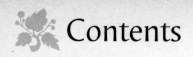

Introducing the diet

The facts and recipes that follow give you all the information you need to make a success of this particular diet. I state 'particular diet' because there are many regimes you could follow to try and alleviate the effects of arthritis. This is the diet that brought me relief some years ago and still prevents my arthritis bothering me.

MARGUERITE PATTEN

WHY DID I CHOOSE THIS DIET?

Because it seemed to me to fit in with my food preferences. I could have decided on a dairy-free diet but I discarded that – I am too fond of cheese and other dairy foods. I like vegetarian dishes but was very disinclined to give up meat, poultry, game and fish.

I read of the extraordinary success achieved by people who followed Dr Giraud W. Campbell's advice, so in 1993 I began my dietary fight against this affliction.

DID I FIND IT DIFFICULT TO KEEP TO THE RULES?

In 1993, when I read through the essential information, I must confess I felt it would be very difficult to follow the diet. However, when I began eating the recommended foods I found it very possible, and as soon as I began to feel a definite improvement in my mobility and a reduction in pain, I knew I was on the right lines. I did not enjoy giving up tea and coffee but discovered many other drinks instead (see page 82).

The diet made me realize how much wheat we eat nowadays – for we enjoy pasta and couscous as well as bread, biscuits, cakes and many other things made with flour.

I love citrus fruits, but I had to forego those for a time, together with alcohol. By 2000, when I began work on my part of this book, many more facts had been discovered about foods that may well affect arthritis, including those vegetables in the nightshade group (outlined on page 57), so these are omitted in the initial meals.

FOR HOW LONG DID I FOLLOW THE INITIAL DIET IN 1993?

I kept to the strict rules for three weeks, then in the fourth week, when I was so much better, I introduced the thing I missed most – oranges. I ate them sparingly and was fine. It was only when I started to have them 'ad lib' that I noticed I had more pain – so that taught me to be careful about citrus fruits.

When writing this book I went back on the diet for a week – it did me good. I followed it implicitly for the second week but introduced tomatoes and had them every day – no adverse effect. I then went on to include aubergines (eggplants), peppers and potatoes – again I was fine. In my case vegetables in the nightshade family do not affect my arthritis.

DO I FOLLOW A STRICT DIET ALL THE TIME?

No, I do not. I could not do my job as a cookery writer, which entails testing, cooking and eating a wide variety of foods, if I ate a strictly limited range of ingredients. Over the years I have found the foods I need to avoid on a regular basis, and adjust my intake accordingly.

In my case I am better if I eat a restricted amount of wheat, so I avoid this entirely where possible. If I do have toast for breakfast, I try not to eat pasta or anything else made with wheat for the rest of the day.

I avoid tea, coffee and wine. From time to time, when I am with friends, I have the odd cup or glass. I enjoy that, but never drink any more that day. I need to curb my love of tall glasses of fresh orange juice. I still drink it, but in much smaller amounts.

Those are **my** results, but **yours** may well be different. The important thing is for **you** to take charge of what you eat, note the results and then act accordingly.

I eat a large amount of fresh fruit and vegetables. I try to buy good-quality organic foods. I do avoid most convenience foods, except for testing purposes. Finally, I treat the foods Jeannette Ewin says should be avoided with respect, and rarely eat them.

Do I ever return to the diet?

Yes, if I have a bad patch then I go back to the strict diet for a few days. When I say a bad patch I mean odd niggles of pain – nothing like as bad as in the pre-1993 days.

I always try and have liver, kidneys or sweetbreads once a week. As I enjoy these foods it is no hardship. Also, I try and keep physically active and watch my weight. After spending a long time at my desk I then try to spend an hour or so gardening or walking to compensate for this.

Do I take supplements?

I have taken cod-liver oil since 1993. Since 2000 I have been buying it combined with fish oils, and take the strong one-a-day capsules.

I drink 300ml/10fl oz/1¼ cups of pasteurized milk every day. The original diet suggests stirring brewers' yeast and black treacle (molasses) into this to make a health drink. I hated it, so I take the brewers' yeast as tablets and a spoonful of black treacle before the milk.

I have never taken any medical tablets, but you must follow your doctor's advice on that matter.

Is my arthritis completely cured?

No. I still have stiffness climbing stairs, but I can live a perfectly normal life, generally without any pain whatsoever. Before I began the diet in 1993 I was badly disabled and had terrible pain.

What would my advice be to anyone who has the first twinge of arthritis?

I would follow the advice in this book, and change to gluten-free bread and breakfast cereals.

The menus

The menus that follow are a guide for the first weeks of your arthritis diet. It is essential to follow the advice from Jeannette Ewin as to the foods to include, and those to avoid, during this initial period.

You can change around the dishes for various days to suit yourself but it is important to include the amount of liver and/or kidney suggested, together with the Health Drink of milk, brewers' yeast and black treacle (molasses) (see page 71).

When you read the menus it may seem an excessive amount of food is being recommended. Remember, while you are finding out just what foods could affect your arthritis, you have to avoid familiar things such as bread, pasta and potatoes, together with ready-prepared breakfast cereals and porridge. These are satisfying and sustaining so you need other foods to take their place. If you have overlooked root vegetables such as celeriac, parsnips, turnips and sweet potatoes in the past include plenty of these in salads and as cooked vegetables. Polenta (which comes from maize) is another satisfying food. You will find a recipe for cooking this on page 170.

Gluten-free breads and pasta are readily available in supermarkets so you could use these from time to time.

If you do feel pangs of hunger do not rush to the biscuit tin, for most biscuits are based upon wheat, oats or other grains. Choose a favourite fruit instead.

I have suggested you include a banana as part of your breakfast each morning, as it is very satisfying. If, by chance, you have no time for a more elaborate meal do at least eat the banana.

What can I drink?

If you are a lover of tea and coffee you will be somewhat unhappy at the thought that these must be avoided completely during the initial stages of your diet. In fact you may well find that your arthritis is better if you avoid or limit these beverages at all times. What can take their place?

Water: you need to drink as much as possible, so make this your first priority. Drink tap or filtered water. Still bottled water is fine, but not carbonated.

Commercial fruit juices: the most readily-available ones are apple (there is a wonderful selection of organic and pure apple juice), grape juice and pineapple juice. Do not drink any form of citrus fruit juice, or tomato juice. Look out for other interesting pure fruit juices.

Home-made fruit and vegetable juices: juice extractors have become very inexpensive and you may find it worthwhile purchasing one so you can make your own juices and have the fun of combining fruits and vegetables to create a range of drinks. These are wonderfully health-giving but do not enjoy them at the expense of *eating* fresh fruits and vegetables – you need these to add fibre to your diet.

Herb teas: look around in specialist shops and supermarkets and you will find an unbelievable range. You can also make your own herb teas from fresh herbs. Even if you do not grow these you can get them in garden centres and supermarkets. Choose those grown in pots, so you have them really freshly-grown, and look for organically grown ones. Wash well in cold water before using.

My favourites are mint and lemon balm. Pick a number of leaves, put them into the cup or mug, crush slightly with a spoon, then add the boiling water. Both of these make refreshing cold teas too. Infuse the leaves in the boiling water, then chill well before straining.

Milk: this is one of the main ingredients of the Health Drink recommended on page 71, but extra milk can be used to make milk shakes (now often known as smoothies) in the liquidizer. Simply blend the milk with fresh fruits of your choice. These become a food as well as a drink and can take the place of a dessert.

There are recommendations about various types of milk on page 60. This information is important if you are allergic to cows' milk.

The first seven days of the diet

I have not given specific vegetables and fruits for these will vary according to the season of the year. Just serve an ample selection at each main meal. But do check the advice on the vegetables and fruits to avoid during this time (see page 57).

Try and eat a good breakfast. If you are not a breakfast eater then have fruit mid-morning. Undoubtedly you will miss drinking tea and coffee at first but you will find alternative suggestions given above.

The main meal could be taken at midday or in the evening, and the lighter meal for lunch or supper. Some of the salads will be suitable as packed meals for workers.

DAY 1	No meals	Just drink plenty of water. Work out how you will cope with this. You may decide to have a day of leisure – rest and read a special book – or you may find it better to plan so much activity that you have no time to think about food.
DAY 2	Breakfast	Selection of fresh fruits, including a banana
	Main meal	Liver with Mixed Herbs (see page 135) with vegetables
		Fresh fruit
	Light meal	Selection of fresh fruits
DAY 3	Breakfast	Boiled egg or Millet Porridge (see page 218)
		Banana
	Main meal	Country Lambs' Kidneys (see page 140) with vegetables
		Fresh fruit
	Light meal	Seafood Stir-fry (see page 120)
		Fresh fruit

Day 4	Breakfast	Poached Herring Roes (see page 128)
		Banana
	Main meal	Chicken Liver Risotto (see page 136) with vegetables
		Fresh fruit
	Light meal	Grilled Goat's Cheese Salad (see page 188)
		Fresh fruit
Day 5	Breakfast	Poached egg on Corn Bread toast (see page 222)
		Banana
	Main meal	Grilled Fish with Cucumber Sauce (see pages 114 and 160) with vegetables
		Fresh fruit
	Light meal	Creamy Liver Pâté with Sweetcorn Salad (see pages 92 and 187)
		Fresh fruit
Day 6	Breakfast	Speedy Blinis (see page 214) filled with goat's cheese
		Banana
	Main meal	Liver Stir-fry (see page 121) with vegetables
		Fresh fruit
	Light meal	Grilled Spiced Sardines (see page 126)
		Fresh fruit
Day 7	Breakfast	Savoury Omelette (see page 172) or Millet Muesli (see page 219)
		Banana
	Main meal	Roast Chicken with Almond Relish (see pages 152 and 168) with vegetables
		Fresh fruit
	Light meal	Liver and Herb Salad (see page 190)
		Fresh fruit

The second seven days of the diet

If you are happy to, you can repeat the dishes recommended for the first seven days. Alternatively, follow the change of menus I have provided below for the second week. Although most dishes are different from those in Week One they are still based on the essential foods: liver, or a suitable alternative, and fish, plus fresh fruits and vegetables in season.

If you have seen a real improvement in your arthritis then follow the advice on pages 73–74 and start to introduce new foods gradually. If there is only very little improvement then I suggest you keep to the basic diet for this second week. Add a soup if you want to make the main meal more sustaining. Always include a selection of vegetables.

Day 8	Breakfast	Scrambled egg on Corn Bread toast (see page 222)
		Banana
	Main meal	Liver Soufflé (see page 138) with vegetables
		Fresh fruit
	Light meal	Lentil Soup (see page 104)
		Roquefort cheese and salad
		Fresh fruit
Day 9	Breakfast	Sautéed Cod's Roe (see page 130)
		Banana
	Main meal	Creamed Sweetbreads (see page 142) with vegetables
		Fresh fruit
	Light meal	Lentil and Pine (Pignolia) Nut Salad (see page 197)
		Fresh fruit

Day 10	Breakfast	Mushroom Omelette (see page 174)
		Banana
	Main meal	Fish Véronique (see page 112) with vegetables
		Fresh fruit
	Light meal	Creamy Liver Pâté with Sweet Potato Salad
		(pages 92 and 194)
		Fresh fruit
Day 11	**Breakfast**	Sautéed Kidneys (see page 141)
		Banana
	Main meal	Grilled Fish with Pesto Sauce (pages 114 and
		162) with vegetables
		Fresh fruit
	Light meal	Bean and Walnut Salad (see page 197)
		Fresh fruit
Day 12	**Breakfast**	Boiled egg and Blinis (see page 212)
		Banana
	Main meal	Grilled Liver with Cucumber Coulis (see
		pages 132 and 161) with vegetables
		Fresh fruit
	Light meal	Thai Fish Cakes (see page 124) with vegetables
		Fresh fruit
Day 13	**Breakfast**	Kedgeree (see page 118)
		Banana
	Main meal	Quail with Blueberry Sauce (see page 156)
		with vegetables
		Fresh fruit
	Light meal	Sautéed Liver (see page 134) with a mixed
		salad
		Fresh fruit

Day 14	Breakfast	Avocado moistened with apple or grape juice or Millet Muesli (see page 219)
		Banana
	Main meal	Special Party Buffet (to show everyone that the diet is interesting as well as beneficial)
		Chicken and Almond Soup (page 102)
		Cucumber and Seafood Dip (see page 94)
		Golden Roquefort Dip (see page 96)
		Mushroom and Liver Salad (see page 192)
		Fresh fruit
	Light meal	Beetroot Soup (see page 100)
		Garlic Mushrooms (see page 180) and a mixed salad
		Fresh fruit

Note: in addition to the recipes covering the initial two weeks of the diet you will find a further wide selection enabling you to continue eating in a way that will maintain your good health.

Following the recipes

The ingredients used in the recipes follow Jeannette Ewin's recommendations about the kinds of foods to eat to combat arthritis. As you will have read on pages 46–51 there are certain foods that it is advisable to omit during the first weeks of the diet, but these may be reintroduced gradually, so you can ascertain just what does – or does not – affect your arthritis.

Whatever foods you buy try to ensure they are organic, and therefore free from pesticides, and that they are as fresh as possible. In a few instances you may choose to buy canned foods to save a long cooking time (as in the case of dried beans). Read the labels carefully to avoid brands that contain additives; drain and wash well.

- Wash all fruits, vegetables, fish, meat, etc. well before using them.
- If you wish to use nuts make certain no-one is allergic to these.

MEASURING THE INGREDIENTS

The ingredients for each recipe are given in metric, imperial and American measures so they are easy to follow. All spoon measures are level.

- A metric teaspoon is equivalent to 5ml.
- A metric tablespoon is equivalent to 15ml.
- American teaspoons are similar in size to metric and imperial ones.
- American tablespoons are slightly smaller than metric and imperial tablespoons, so an allowance for this is made in the American column. Where tablespoons are mentioned in the method, the American equivalent is given in brackets.
- An American cup is the equivalent of 226.8ml (8fl oz).
- Metric measures are adjusted slightly to give amounts that are easy to measure or weigh.
- Always follow one set of measurements and not a mixture.

OVEN SETTINGS

The oven settings are given for electricity and gas but in case any readers have cookers without settings the following information will be helpful.

DESCRIPTION	CELSIUS (°C)	FAHRENHEIT (°F)	GAS MARK (NO)
very cool	110–130	225–250	1/4–1/2
cool/slow	140–150	275–300	1–2
warm	160–170	325	3
moderate	180	350	4
moderately hot	190	375	5
fairly hot	200	400	6
hot	220	425	7
very hot	230–240	450–475	8–9

A fan oven or fan-assisted (convection) oven should be set at a slightly lower temperature than an ordinary oven. A general recommendation is given in the recipes but it is wise to check with your manufacturer's handbook too.

USING A MICROWAVE OVEN

In some recipes it is suggested you could use a microwave oven. As these vary a great deal according to the output and the model, check the food from time to time during the cooking process.

It is advisable to allow a few minutes' standing time after the food comes out of the microwave before serving.

SEASONING

It is recommended that sea salt is used, for this contains valuable minerals.

Pepper, like all spices, deteriorates with storage, especially when ready-ground, therefore it is wise to buy small amounts of whole peppercorns and use these in a pepper mill so they are ground each time you need pepper. Most recipes state black pepper but occasionally you will see white mentioned. This is where the dish is light in colour and therefore white pepper is a better choice.

QUANTITIES IN THE RECIPES

Most dishes are planned to serve all the family, generally assumed to be four people. This is because everyone will benefit from the healthy food and I hope they will find the dishes enjoyable as well as nutritious.

Obviously people not suffering from arthritis can add extra ingredients, such as tomatoes and potatoes, etc. to the basic dish if they wish to.

In a few fish recipes, in omelettes, and most liver recipes quantities are given for one person only. In the case of liver, there are two reasons for this. First: not everyone has to eat the regular quantity of liver given in the initial diet – although they may wish to do so. Second: cooked liver does not improve by being kept waiting, so if members of the family are likely to be a little late, it is better to cook it for each person separately. Fortunately the cooking times and method are quick and easy, so that should not be a problem.

Creamy Liver Pâté

The addition of cream in the recipe below gives a more mellow taste to the liver so that it will appeal to most people – even those who are not over-fond of this meat. It is a good basic recipe which can be varied in many ways: you can make it with calves' liver, lambs' liver or chicken livers.

When cooking liver (pages 131–135) you could increase the quantity and mince or process some, then add a little cream and/or melted butter with a crushed garlic clove and chopped herbs to turn it into a very quickly prepared pâté.

Ingredients   SERVES 6–8 AS A STARTER OR 4 AS PART OF A MAIN COURSE

METRIC (IMPERIAL)	AMERICAN
2 teaspoons olive oil	2 teaspoons
2 small shallots or spring onions (scallions), chopped	2
450g (1lb) liver, sliced	1lb
115g (4oz) pork, preferably from fillet	¼lb
2 teaspoons finely chopped sage leaves	2 teaspoons
2 small eggs, beaten	2
3 tablespoons meat stock (bouillon) (see page 99)	3¾ tablespoons
150ml (5fl oz) double (heavy) cream	⅔ cup
sea salt and freshly ground black pepper to taste	
1 teaspoon prepared English or Dijon mustard	1 teaspoon

Method

1 Preheat the oven to 160°C/325°F/Gas Mark 3 or 150°C for a fan (convection) oven. Grease a 900ml (1½ pint) terrine tin or ovenproof container.

2 Heat the olive oil, then add the shallots or spring onions. Turn in the oil for about 4 minutes, then mix with the liver and pork.

3 Put the mixture through a mincer or into a food processor and mince (grind) or chop to the desired texture. If you require a very smooth texture do this twice. If you are using a food processor be careful that you do not over-process, for this makes the meat sticky. Mix in the remaining ingredients.

4 Spoon into the prepared container and press firmly down (this helps the pâté to turn out well). Cover with a lid or foil.

5 Stand in a tin half filled with warm water (a bain-marie) and cook for 1½ hours. Allow to cool, then turn out and serve portions with salad. As you cannot have ordinary toast while on the initial diet, rice cakes are a good accompaniment.

Variations

❋ For a pâté with a stronger taste omit the cream and use 6 (7½) extra tablespoons of stock.

❋ If you have discovered that you can eat citrus fruits, add 2 teaspoons of finely grated lemon zest to give extra flavour to the mixture.

❋ *Millet Liver Pâté:* millet gives an interesting taste and texture to the pâté and also adds extra food value. Take the 3 (3¾) tablespoons stock given in the recipe, heat to boiling point and pour over 3 (3¾) tablespoons of millet. Allow to stand for at least 10 minutes, then add to the other ingredients after they have been minced (ground) or placed in the food processor, see step 3. Continue as in the recipe.

Freezing

Pâtés tend to lose much of their smooth texture in freezing – they become drier and crumbly. This mixture can be frozen for up to 2 weeks without being spoiled.

Cucumber and Seafood Dip

If you find eating salads regularly quite difficult then try combining salad ingredients with an interesting dip. This can be served in a bowl surrounded by a selection of crudités (raw salad ingredients), or you can spoon individual portions of the dip into small bowls and arrange the crudités on a plate. The following could be served as part of a party buffet or as a first course, light lunch or supper dish.

Ingredients

SERVES 4–6

METRIC (IMPERIAL)	AMERICAN
4 tablespoons cucumber, peeled and grated	5 tablespoons
225g (8oz) crabmeat	½lb
175g (6oz) peeled prawns (shelled shrimp), finely chopped	1 cup
3 tablespoons Mayonnaise (see page 166)	3¾ tablespoons
1 tablespoon lemon grass stalk, finely chopped	1 tablespoon
1 tablespoon finely chopped fennel bulb	1¼ tablespoons
sea salt and freshly ground black pepper to taste	
yoghurt to bind	

For the crudités
sticks of carrot, celery, cucumber and courgette (zucchini)

Method

1 Combine all the ingredients except the yoghurt. Mix well so you have a thick, smooth consistency.
2 Gradually add enough yoghurt to give a mixture like thick whipped cream. Taste and adjust the seasoning.

Variations

* If you find you can have a certain amount of citrus fruits use lemon juice instead of lemon grass.
* Flavour the mixture with chopped fresh herbs such as mint, thyme or rosemary.
* Sticks of red, green and yellow (bell) peppers are ideal crudités, if you find you are not allergic to nightshade vegetables.
* *Avocado and Seafood Dip:* substitute the flesh from 1 large or 2 small avocados for the cucumber.

Do not freeze

Golden Roquefort Dip

This is a dip you can make while on the initial diet. Based on delicious Roquefort cheese, sweetcorn and eggs, it is both nutritious and appetizing. Serve it with crudités, as on page 94, and rice cakes. These are obtainable from most health food stores and supermarkets.

Ingredients

SERVES 4–6

METRIC (IMPERIAL)	AMERICAN
1 corn cob	1
sea salt and freshly ground black pepper to taste	
2 large eggs, hard-boiled (hard-cooked)	2
175g (6oz) Roquefort cheese, crumbled	1 cup
3 tablespoons Mayonnaise (see page 166)	3¾ tablespoons
2 tablespoons finely chopped spring onions (scallions) or chives	2½ tablespoons
double (heavy) cream or yoghurt to bind	
few drops balsamic or other vinegar, optional to taste	
crudités as page 94	

Method

1 Strip away the outer leaves from the corn cob and put the cob into boiling water. Do not add salt at this stage as it tends to prevent the corn becoming tender; add a little towards the end of the cooking time.
2 Strip the kernels from the cob into a bowl; season lightly.
3 Remove the shells from the eggs and chop the whites and yolks separately. Mix the whites with the sweetcorn, cheese, mayonnaise and spring onions or chives.
4 Gradually stir in enough cream or yoghurt to give the dip the consistency of whipped cream. Taste and add a little vinegar if desired.
5 Spoon into a suitable bowl or bowls and top with the chopped egg yolks just before serving. Surround with crudités and rice cakes.

Variations

- When you are introducing other foods into the diet you could use Stilton, Gorgonzola or other blue cheeses instead of Roquefort.
- Finely chopped sun-dried tomatoes add both flavour and colour but avoid these for the first two weeks of the diet.

Do not freeze

Making Stock

Several recipes in this book mention stock (bouillon). This is the liquid that will give the dish a really good flavour. It is possible to purchase ready-prepared stocks in various convenient forms (cube, liquid or powder). However, during the initial stages of your diet you are trying to avoid ready-made products, so it is sensible to make your own stock. The conventional method of making stock is given below, but you could also use a microwave or a covered casserole in the oven for this purpose.

If it is not possible to make stock, buy additive-free stock cubes or powders.

In each of the recipes below the amount of stock made will be about 600ml (1 pint/2½ cups). After cooking, strain the stock through a fine sieve.

Chicken Stock
Simmer the carcass of a cooked chicken with 1 or 2 chopped onions, 1 chopped carrot and 1 or 2 chopped celery sticks in 1.5 litres (2½ pints/4¼ cups) of water. Add sprigs of thyme, 1 or 2 fresh bay leaves, sea salt and freshly ground black pepper. Allow it to simmer for 1¼–1½ hours. To give a stronger-tasting stock add a portion of uncooked chicken.

Fish Stock
This is made by simmering the heads, skins and bones of fish and/or the shells of seafood like lobster or prawns. Put about 450g (1lb) of fish trimmings into a pan with 900ml (1½ pints/3¾ cups) of water. Add 1 chopped onion, 1 chopped carrot, 1 chopped celery stick, a good sprig of chervil or parsley, a sprig of thyme, sea salt and freshly ground black pepper. Simmer for 25–30 minutes and strain after cooking.

Meat Stock

Use about 450g (1lb) of beef or lamb bones*, together with similar vegetables, herbs and seasonings to those used in the recipe for Chicken Stock. You will obtain a richer flavour and colour if the bones and vegetables are first browned in a pan in a small amount of oil. Allow 1.8 litres (3 pints) or 7½ cups of water and simmer for at least 2 hours.

Vegetable Stock

Use about 450g (1lb) of mixed vegetables to 1.2 litres (2 pints/5 cups) of water. Add herbs that will give the appropriate flavour to the dishes in which the stock will be used. Season lightly with sea salt and freshly ground black pepper. The cooking time will vary according to the size of the vegetables. If finely chopped, allow about 30 minutes; 40 minutes if in larger pieces. Do not overcook.

Freezing

Allow the stock to cool then remove any fat from the top of the liquid. Pack into suitable containers; allow 2cm (¾ inch) headroom as stock expands when frozen.

*Uncooked bones make a stronger-flavoured stock but bones from cooked meat can be used.

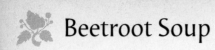

Beetroot Soup

If you have a sweet tooth include plenty of beetroot (beets) in your salads as it has a wonderful natural sweetness. It is also an excellent vegetable to serve hot, or to make into a soup. This soup is equally good hot or cold.

Ingredients

SERVES 4

METRIC (IMPERIAL)	AMERICAN
1 medium red (mild) onion, finely chopped	1 medium
600ml (1 pint) chicken or vegetable stock (bouillon) (see pages 98–99)	2½ cups
225g (8oz) cooked beetroot (weight when peeled and chopped)	½lb
300ml (10fl oz) yoghurt	1¼ cups
sea salt and freshly ground black pepper to taste	

To garnish
chopped watercress leaves

Method

1 Put the onion and stock into a saucepan, bring just to the boil, then lower the heat and simmer for 10 minutes.
2 Add the beetroot, then liquidize the mixture.
3 *To serve hot:* bring the soup just to boiling point then whisk in the yoghurt and heat gently; do not allow to boil again. Season to taste. Garnish and serve.
4 *To serve cold:* chill the liquidized mixture well and whisk in the yoghurt and seasoning just before serving. Garnish and serve.

Variation

🌿 Increase the amount of watercress leaves and liquidize some of these with the beetroot mixture.

Do not freeze

Chicken and Almond Soup

Almonds were traditionally used as a thickening instead of flour, so this tasty soup fits well into the basic diet.

Ingredients

METRIC (IMPERIAL)	AMERICAN
1 small onion, chopped	1
900ml (1½ pints) chicken stock (bouillon) (see page 98)	3¾ cups
1 chicken breast	1
sea salt and freshly ground black pepper to taste	
50g (2oz) ground almonds	½ cup

To garnish

2 small eggs, hard-boiled (hard-cooked)	2
2 tablespoons chopped parsley	2½ tablespoons

Method

1 Put the onion, stock and chicken breast into a saucepan, season lightly, then cover the pan and simmer for 30 minutes.

2 Stir in the ground almonds, then tip the soup into a liquidizer or food processor. Process to a smooth purée.

3 Return to the pan and reheat gently. Meanwhile, shell the eggs and chop the whites and yolks separately. Stir the whites into the soup.

4 Pour the soup into individual soup bowls and top with the chopped egg yolks and parsley.

Variation

✿ A little double (heavy) cream can be stirred into the soup just before serving.

Freezing

The soup can be frozen at the end of step 2.

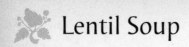

Lentil Soup

I use the small split orange lentils for this soup as they give it a good colour. They need no soaking and become tender quite quickly, so do not overcook the soup as you need to retain the fresh flavour.

Ingredients

METRIC (IMPERIAL)	AMERICAN
1½ tablespoons sunflower oil	scant 2 tablespoons
2 medium onions, finely chopped	2
1 garlic clove, chopped	1
2 small carrots, thinly sliced	2
600ml (1 pint) water	2½ cups
225g (8oz) lentils	1 cup
1 small dessert apple, peeled, cored and finely chopped	1
bouquet garni (bunch of parsley, sage, thyme and coriander tied with cotton)	
sea salt and freshly ground black pepper to taste	
1 tablespoon cornflour (cornstarch)	1¼ tablespoons
300ml (10fl oz) or as required milk	1¼ cups or as required

To garnish
chopped parsley or coriander (cilantro)

Method

1 Heat the oil in a large saucepan, add the onions and cook gently for 5 minutes. Stir in the garlic and carrots and cook for another 2 minutes.

2 Pour the water into the saucepan and bring to the boil. Add the lentils, apple, bouquet garni and seasoning to taste.

3 Bring the liquid back to the boil, stir briskly, then lower the heat and cover the pan. Simmer gently for 45 minutes. Remove the bouquet garni.

4 Mix the cornflour with the milk, pour into the saucepan and stir over a low heat until the mixture thickens.

5 Pour the soup into a liquidizer or food processor and process until very smooth. Return to the saucepan and heat. If it is a little too thick add more milk. Taste and adjust the seasoning.

6 Serve the soup topped with a generous amount of parsley or coriander.

Freezing
Cook to the end of step 5, cool then pack and freeze. Remember to leave 2cm (¾ inch) headroom in the container.

Indonesian Chicken Soup

This is so filling it could be described as a meal in a soup. It is also packed with flavour. Leave out the canned water chestnuts while you are on the strict diet and use pine (pignolia) nuts or chopped, blanched almonds instead to give an interesting texture. Omit the lime juice if avoiding citrus fruits.

Ingredients

SERVES 4–6

METRIC (IMPERIAL)	AMERICAN
2 tablespoons groundnut or sunflower oil	2½ tablespoons
2 medium onions, finely chopped	2
2 garlic cloves, finely chopped	2
1 tablespoon grated root ginger	1¼ tablespoons
2 chicken breasts, finely chopped	2
1.2 litres (2 pints) chicken stock (bouillon) (see page 98)	5 cups
1 tablespoon thinly sliced lemon grass	1¼ tablespoons
150ml (5fl oz) coconut milk	⅔ cup
2 canned water chestnuts, finely diced, optional – see above	2
sea salt and freshly ground black pepper to taste	
50g (2oz) fresh bean sprouts	1 cup
1 tablespoon lime juice, optional – see above	1¼ tablespoons
2 tablespoons chopped coriander (cilantro)	2½ tablespoons

Method

1 Heat the oil in a saucepan, add the onions and cook for 5 minutes, then stir in the garlic, ginger and chicken. Continue stirring over a moderate heat for a further 5 minutes.
2 Add the stock and lemon grass, bring to the boil, then lower the heat, cover the pan and simmer for 10 minutes.
3 Pour in the coconut milk and add the water chestnuts, a little seasoning and the bean sprouts. Simmer for 3–4 minutes then stir in the lime juice and half the coriander. Adjust the seasoning and serve topped with the remaining coriander.

Variation

❀ To make an even more sustaining soup, top with chopped hard-boiled (hard-cooked) eggs as well as coriander.

Do not freeze

Liver and Mushroom Soup

This soup can be made within a very short time if you have the chicken stock (bouillon) available. The method of making this is given on page 98.

Ingredients

METRIC (IMPERIAL)	AMERICAN
1 litre (1¾ pints) chicken stock (bouillon) (see page 98)	scant 4½ cups
1 medium bunch spring onions (scallions)	1 medium bunch
350g (12oz) mushrooms (can be mixed types), wiped	¾lb
sea salt and freshly ground black pepper to taste	
175g (6oz) cooked liver (see page 132), finely diced	¾ cup

To garnish

2 tablespoons chopped coriander (cilantro)	2½ tablespoons

Method

1 Pour the chicken stock into a saucepan. Remove the green ends from the spring onions and add the white bulbs to the pan with the whole mushrooms.
2 Bring the stock to the boil, add a little seasoning, then lower the heat and cover the pan. Simmer steadily for 20 minutes. Remove from the heat and add the liver.
3 Ladle the soup into a liquidizer or food processor. Process to a smooth purée.
4 Return to the pan, check the seasoning and add a little more if required. Bring just to the boil, then pour into individual soup bowls, garnish with the coriander and serve.

Variation

❈ *Kidney and Mushroom Soup:* use the same amount of kidneys (cooked as on page 140) instead of liver.

Freezing

The soup can be frozen at the end of step 3. Remember to leave 2cm (³/₄ inch) headroom.

Cod with Pineapple and Cucumber

This dish is perfect for those avoiding citrus fruits, as its refreshing flavour is provided not by lemon or lime but by pineapple. The quantities are for a single person. If cooking for more people wrap each portion of fish separately.

Ingredients

SERVES 1

METRIC (IMPERIAL)	AMERICAN
1 teaspoon olive oil	1 teaspoon
50g (2oz) cucumber, peeled and thinly sliced	½ cup
3 teaspoons chopped mint	3 teaspoons
sea salt and freshly ground black pepper to taste	
2 slices fresh pineapple, 2cm (¾ inch) thick	2 slices
1 portion cod cutlet, 2.5cm (1 inch) thick	1 portion

Method

1   Preheat the oven to 190°C/375°F/Gas Mark 5 or 180°C for a fan (convection) oven. Cut a square of foil sufficiently large to envelop the ingredients, and brush the middle with the oil.

2   Place half the cucumber on the foil, then add half the mint and a little seasoning.

3   Cut away the outer skin and centre hard core from the pineapple and place one ring over the cucumber. Add the fish.

4   Cover the fish with the second ring of pineapple then with the remaining cucumber, mint and more seasoning. Fold the foil to enclose the ingredients.

5   Place on a baking sheet and cook for 30 minutes. Open the foil carefully, as steam builds up inside. Serve with a crisp salad or lightly cooked vegetables.

Variations

❋ Use 4 teaspoons of finely chopped lemon grass instead of, or with, the mint.

❋ Cod is becoming increasingly scarce so you may want to use another white fish such as haddock.

Do not freeze

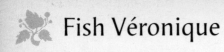

Fish Véronique

This is a version of one of the great classic fish dishes. Originally it was based upon sole, but plaice or whiting are good alternatives. The fish needs to be filleted and then skinned. Use the bones and skin to make your fish stock (bouillon) (see page 98). The classic fish recipes almost invariably use wine with fish stock, so I have substituted a little pure grape juice.

Ingredients

SERVES 4

METRIC (IMPERIAL)	AMERICAN
150g (5oz) black or white grapes	scant 1 cup
4 large or 8 small fish fillets, without skin and bones	4 large or 8 small
300ml (10fl oz) fish stock (bouillon) (see page 98)	1¼ cups
2 tablespoons grape juice	2½ tablespoons
sea salt and freshly ground white pepper to taste	

For the sauce

25g (1oz) butter	2 tablespoons
15g (½oz) cornflour (cornstarch)	1 tablespoon
150ml (5fl oz) double (heavy) cream	⅔ cup

To garnish

black and/or white grapes
fennel leaves

Method

1 Preheat the oven to 200°C/400°F/Gas Mark 6 or 190°C for a fan (convection) oven.

2 If the grapes are seedless just slit them so the juice will run out during cooking. If they contain seeds halve the grapes and remove them. The grapes could be peeled but this is not essential.

3 Place the grapes on the fillets of fish, then roll up to enclose the fruit. Secure with wooden cocktail sticks (tooth picks) and lay in a large ovenproof dish.

4 Mix the fish stock and grape juice, pour over the fish and add a little seasoning. Cover the dish and bake for 25 minutes or until the fish is just tender. Carefully lift the fillets on to another dish, cover and keep hot.

5 Strain 250ml (8fl oz/1 cup) of the stock from the dish.

6 Heat the butter in a small saucepan, stir in the cornflour, then gradually add the fish liquid and whisk as the mixture comes to the boil and thickens. Stir in the cream and continue stirring until smooth; season to taste.

7 Remove the cocktail sticks and coat the fish with the sauce. Garnish with grapes and fennel leaves. Rings of cooked fennel bulb and broccoli florets are good accompaniments.

Do not freeze

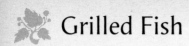

Grilled Fish

Grilling (broiling) is a very healthy way of cooking fish. Only a small amount of fat is required, just enough to keep the fish beautifully moist as it cooks. Because grilling is a fast method of cooking, the fish retains maximum flavour and a moist texture. Always preheat the grill before putting the fish under it.

I do not specify the choice of fish in the first menus but leave that to you. Do not be too conservative in your choice. As well as white fish, such as sole, plaice, cod and halibut, remember good oily fish, like salmon (not in the initial diet) herring and trout; and the modern favourites, fresh tuna and swordfish. Always buy the freshest fish possible.

Ingredients

SERVES 4

METRIC (IMPERIAL)	**AMERICAN**
4 portions fish	4 portions
sea salt and freshly ground white or black pepper to taste	
50g (2oz) butter, melted; or olive oil	¼ cup

To garnish
Cucumber Sauce (see page 160)
parsley and watercress

Method

1 Preheat the grill (broiler) well. Wash the fish thoroughly in cold water and pat dry with paper towels. To save the grill pan picking up fishy flavours line it with foil (discard after cooking).

2 Season the fish and also add seasoning to the butter. Brush the foil with a very little butter, place the fish on top and brush the top of the fish with butter.

3 Cook thin fillets of fish for 4–5 minutes and do not turn them over. Cook thicker fish fillets and cutlets for 8–10 minutes; turn halfway through the cooking time and brush with more seasoned butter. Whole fish or solid fish slices (often known as steaks) may need up to 15 minutes. Cook these on a fairly high heat on each side, reducing it slightly for the last few minutes.

4 Check that the fish is cooked by piercing the thickest part with the tip of a knife; the flesh should look opaque, not translucent. Garnish and serve.

Flavouring Fish

- White fish is best with the more delicate flavourings. As you are not using lemon or lime juice at the beginning of the diet, substitute crushed and chopped lemon grass or chopped lemon balm leaves. Parsley and other herbs, such as fennel, dill or coriander (cilantro) all blend well with white fish. If you find you are not allergic to citrus fruits then be generous with lime, lemon and orange zest and juice.
- White fish also goes well with the flavour of bananas. Fry fillets of fish in a little butter and oil with some sliced bananas. Add finely chopped chives as well as seasoning.
- Oily fish can have more robust flavourings such as grated root ginger, chilli powder, garlic and various kinds of mustard.
- Meaty fish like tuna and swordfish are best marinated before cooking.

To make a marinade for 4 portions of fish:

1 Mix together 2 (2½) tablespoons olive oil, 2 teaspoons sesame seed oil, 2 (2½) tablespoons balsamic vinegar, 1 crushed garlic clove, sea salt and freshly ground black pepper.
2 Place the fish in the marinade and leave for 1 hour. Do not leave for any longer or the marinade may make the fish over-tender.
3 Lift the fish out of the marinade, drain well and grill as instructed on page 115. Baste with the marinade during cooking.

Do not freeze

Herbed Baked Fish

Do not be sparing with the fresh herbs used in this dish. They add a splendid flavour to any white fish, and also to fresh salmon.

Ingredients

SERVES 4

METRIC (IMPERIAL)	AMERICAN
2 tablespoons olive oil	2½ tablespoons
6–8 small courgettes (zucchini), thinly sliced	6–8
1 large bunch spring onions (scallions), chopped	1 large bunch
2 tablespoons chopped parsley	2½ tablespoons
1 tablespoon chopped coriander (cilantro)	1¼ tablespoon
1 tablespoon chopped basil	1¼ tablespoon
3 tablespoons fish stock (bouillon) (see page 98)	3¾ tablespoons
4 portions white fish or salmon	4 portions

Method

1 Brush a large ovenproof dish with a little of the oil. Arrange the courgettes in a neat layer in the dish, then top with the spring onions, half the herbs and half the stock.

2 Place the fish on top and cover with the remaining stock, then the last of the herbs. Finally, spoon the remaining oil evenly over the ingredients. Cover the dish with a lid or foil.

3 Preheat the oven to 190°C/375°F/Gas Mark 5 or 180°C for a fan (convection) oven. Bake thin fillets of fish for 15–20 minutes and thicker cutlets for 25–30 minutes.

4 Serve with a crisp green salad.

Do not freeze

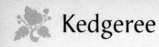

Kedgeree

Although it is famous as a breakfast dish, kedgeree could be served at any time of the day. Its association with India is indicated by the optional use of a small amount of curry powder. The version below is different from the classic one, for that is based upon smoked haddock and, as you will have read, smoked or salted fish and meats of all kinds should be avoided. That does not make this kedgeree less interesting, but gives you more scope to be imaginative in your choice of fish. I have suggested cod in the main recipe but given further suggestions too.

Kedgeree is practical for breakfast as the rice and fish are already cooked, so it is simply a matter of putting these together. Cook the rice in your favourite way and poach the cod in seasoned water. To give the weight of cooked rice in the recipe you need about 115g (4oz) or a good ½ cup of raw rice.

Ingredients

SERVES 4

METRIC (IMPERIAL)	AMERICAN
2 large eggs	2
50g (2oz) butter	¼ cup
1 teaspoon or to taste curry powder, optional	1 teaspoon or to taste
350g (12oz) cooked long grain rice, preferably brown	good 2 cups
350g (12oz) cooked cod, free from bones and skin, broken into large flakes	¾lb
2 tablespoons single (light) cream or milk	2½ tablespoons
sea salt and cayenne pepper to taste	

Method

1 Hard-boil (hard-cook) the eggs. Shell them, then chop the yolks and whites separately.
2 Heat the butter in a saucepan, stir in the curry powder, if using, then add the rice and fish together with the cream or milk. Stir over a medium heat until piping hot.
3 Add the egg white and any seasoning required. Spoon on to a large hot dish or individual plates and garnish with the egg yolk.

Variations

✿ Often fried onion rings were added with the egg yolks as a garnish but they are less suitable for breakfast time.
✿ *Scallop Kedgeree:* lightly fry 6–8 large (king) scallops, then slice thinly and use instead of cooked fish. Save this dish until after the initial diet.
✿ Use any other firm fish, such as halibut or monkfish.
✿ Chopped fresh parsley or thyme can be added to give flavour and colour to the dish.

Do not freeze

Seafood Stir-fry

This is an excellent way of cooking a complete meal in a large frying pan (skillet) or wok. The vegetables should be young and cut into small pieces so they cook quickly and the fish sufficiently firm in texture not to break up with stirring. Makes of soy sauce vary, so check that you are using a brand that does not include a lot of additives. The quality of the stock (bouillon) makes a lot of difference to the success of the dish.

For the first part of the diet use all white fish and no prawns (shrimp). Defrost and dry frozen cooked prawns so that they are firm when added to the pan.

Ingredients
SERVES 4

METRIC (IMPERIAL)	AMERICAN
3 teaspoons cornflour (cornstarch)	3 teaspoons
sea salt and freshly ground white pepper to taste	
450–675g (1–1½lb) firm white fish, such as monkfish, cut into narrow strips, free from skin and bone	1–1½lb
2 tablespoons sunflower or groundnut oil	2½ tablespoons
115g (4oz) mangetout (snow peas)	¼lb
115g (4oz) baby sweetcorn, halved	¼lb
2 or 3 young carrots, cut into narrow strips	2 or 3
150ml (5fl oz) fish stock (bouillon) (see page 98)	⅔ cup
1 tablespoon rice vinegar	1¼ tablespoons
2 teaspoons soy sauce	2 teaspoons
1 teaspoon grated root ginger, optional	1 teaspoon
1 teaspoon, or to taste honey	1 teaspoon, or to taste
175g (6oz) peeled prawns (shrimp)	1 cup

Method

1 Put half the cornflour, with a little seasoning, on to a plate. Add the fish strips and stir around gently until dusted with the cornflour.

2 Heat the oil in a large frying pan (skillet) or wok. Add the coated fish and sauté for about 3 minutes or until delicately brown on the outside. Lift out of the pan with a fish slice or perforated spoon and place on a plate.

3 Stir in the vegetables and continue stirring over the heat for about 5 minutes or until nearly cooked. They should retain a firm texture.

4 Mix the remaining cornflour with the stock, vinegar, soy sauce, ginger and honey. Pour into the pan and stir until the mixture forms a sauce. Return the white fish to the pan and stir over a moderate heat until tender. Add the prawns together with any seasoning required. Heat for 1–2 minutes and serve with cooked brown rice.

Variations

❋ Add other vegetables, such as florets of cauliflower or broccoli or tender green beans – these could be cut into 5cm (2 inch) lengths.

❋ *Chicken Stir-fry:* use strips of uncooked chicken instead of fish. Coat, then cook for about 5 minutes at step 2. Prawns may be an unusual accompaniment to chicken but they blend well together so these could be included. If the prawns are omitted use 450g (1lb) of chicken breast or leg meat – weight without skin and bones. Use chicken stock instead of fish stock (see page 98).

❋ *Liver Stir-fry:* use chicken livers instead of strips of fish. You will need about 450g (1lb) to serve four people. Do not coat with cornflour, simply season very lightly, then sauté for 2 minutes at step 2. Continue as in the recipe but exclude the prawns. Broccoli, shiitake mushrooms, asparagus tips and baby courgettes are particularly good with the liver instead of mangetout, sweetcorn and carrots. Stir-fry the vegetables first then add to the liver when it is almost cooked. Use meat or chicken stock instead of fish stock (see pages 98–99).

Do not freeze

Mussels in Cream Sauce

Green-lipped mussels have become well known as one of the foods that may benefit people suffering from arthritis. Sadly these are not found throughout the world but only in New Zealand. However, they are exported, both fresh or pre-cooked and frozen. Ordinary mussels are more readily available and make a nutritious and very appetizing dish.

Ingredients

METRIC (IMPERIAL)	AMERICAN
2 litres (3½ pints) fresh mussels	8½ cups
1–2 garlic cloves, chopped (optional)	1–2
1 medium onion, finely chopped	1
1 small bunch parsley	1 small bunch
250ml (8fl oz) water	1 cup
sea salt and black pepper to taste	
1–2 lemon grass stalks, chopped	1–2
300ml (10fl oz) double (heavy) cream	1¼ cups

To garnish

2 tablespoons chopped parsley	2½ tablespoons
1 tablespoon chopped coriander (cilantro)	1 tablespoon

Method

1 Wash the mussels in plenty of cold water to remove the grit. If you have managed to obtain green-lipped mussels there is virtually no grit on them. Pull or cut away the small weed (the beard) you may find on some of the shells.

2 Check carefully for any mussels that are open. Tap them firmly, and if the shells fail to close discard them.

3 Put the mussels, garlic (if using), onion, bunch of parsley and water into a large saucepan. Add a very little seasoning, then the lemon grass.

4 Heat steadily for 4–5 minutes or until the shells are open. Do not overcook for that toughens the flesh. Strain, reserving the liquid.

5 Check carefully again and if any mussels remain closed discard them. For this dish the mussels can be removed from the shells.

6 Heat the strained liquid, add the cream, bring to simmering point and heat slowly, stirring, until thickened. Put in the mussels and cook for 2 minutes only. Taste and adjust the seasoning. Top with the chopped parsley and coriander and serve with cooked rice and a selection of vegetables or a salad.

Variations

* If using ready-cooked, frozen, green-lipped mussels defrost at room temperature, then remove from the shells. These mussels are larger than the more familiar type so you need fewer. Use fish stock (see page 98) or water and heat this with the mussel shells and ingredients given in step 3 for 5 minutes, strain and continue with steps 5 and 6.

* If you find you can include citrus fruit in your diet add a little lemon juice to the liquid instead of, or as well as, lemon grass. If you are eating tomatoes add 2 (2½) tablespoons finely diced sun-dried tomatoes at step 6.

* Instead of straining the stock at step 4 simply remove the bunch of parsley and retain the chopped ingredients.

Do not freeze

Thai Fish Cakes

This recipe uses a small amount of prepared curry paste so it should be made when you have completed your initial diet. Any firm white fish is suitable for this dish.

Ingredients

SERVES 4

METRIC (IMPERIAL)	AMERICAN
350g (12oz) firm white fish (weight without bones or skin)	¾lb
2 teaspoons vegetable oil	2 teaspoons
1 shallot or small onion, chopped	1
1 garlic clove	1
1 teaspoon Thai green curry paste	1 teaspoon
2 tablespoons, or as required fish stock (bouillon) (see page 98)	2½ tablespoons, or as required
1 tablespoon chopped coriander (cilantro)	1¼ tablespoons
1 egg, whisked	1
sea salt and freshly ground black pepper to taste	
1 tablespoon, or as required cornflour (cornstarch)	1¼ tablespoons, or as required

For coating and frying

1 tablespoon cornflour (cornstarch)	1¼ tablespoons
2 tablespoons vegetable oil	2½ tablespoons

Method

1   Process the fish lightly (over-processing makes the cakes rubbery) and put on one side. Heat the oil in a frying pan (skillet), add the shallot or onion and garlic and fry gently for 4 minutes.

2   Stir in the curry paste, blend with the other ingredients and heat for 1 minute. Stir in the fish and mix well. Gradually add enough fish stock plus the coriander and egg to give a fairly soft mixture; season to taste.

3   Stir in enough cornflour to make the mixture easy to handle. Do not be too generous with the cornflour. If the mixture is a little over-soft chill for a time in the refrigerator. The fish cakes should never be too dry.

4   Put the coating cornflour on to a plate and mix with a little salt and pepper. Form the fish mixture into about 12 balls, or round cakes if more convenient, then roll in the cornflour. It is easier to fry them if they are chilled for a short time.

5   Heat the oil and fry the fish cakes for 5 minutes, turning them until evenly browned.

Freezing

Do not freeze for longer than 2 weeks. The fish cakes tend to lose their moist texture.

Grilled Spiced Sardines

Fresh sardines are both plentiful and delicious. They make a very good light meal served with a salad or lightly cooked vegetables. Choose really plump fish and use as soon as possible after purchase.

Ingredients

SERVES 4

METRIC (IMPERIAL)	AMERICAN
12 large fresh sardines	12
50g (2oz) butter	¼ cup
¼ teaspoon or to taste chilli powder	¼ teaspoon or to taste
¼ teaspoon ground cumin	¼ teaspoon
2 tablespoons finely chopped coriander (cilantro)	2½ tablespoons
2 tablespoons chopped parsley	2½ tablespoons
2 teaspoons balsamic or sherry vinegar	2 teaspoons
1 tablespoon sunflower oil	1¼ tablespoons
sea salt and freshly ground black pepper to taste	

To garnish
coriander (cilantro) leaves

Method

1   Cut off the sardine heads, then split along the stomach of each fish and open out until flat; carefully remove the intestines. If you wish you can take out the backbones (see below). Rinse in cold water and dry well.

2   Mix the butter with the chilli powder, cumin, coriander, parsley and vinegar. Spread over the inside of each fish then fold so the fish look whole again.

3   Preheat the grill (broiler) and place a sheet of foil over the grid. Brush the foil and the fish with the oil and season to taste.

4   Cook for about 10 minutes. There is no need to turn the fish. Garnish and serve hot.

Variations

* Allow 1 large or 2 small herrings per person instead of the sardines. You will need double the amount of filling for herrings.

* Use cayenne pepper instead of chilli powder.

* To bone the fish: turn the split fish skin side uppermost, run your finger down the backbone very firmly, turn over and you will find you can gently lift away the backbone.

Do not freeze

Poached Herring Roes

Herring roes, especially the soft kind, are exceptionally easy to digest, and make a nourishing dish for breakfast or for a light snack. Their creamy texture makes them especially good served on toast.

Ingredients

METRIC (IMPERIAL)	AMERICAN
450g (1lb) soft herring roes	1lb
4 tablespoons milk	5 tablespoons
25g (1oz) butter	2 tablespoons
sea salt and freshly ground white pepper to taste	

To garnish
paprika or cayenne pepper

Method

1 The herring roes can be cooked in a saucepan but they keep a better shape, and look more attractive, if they are cooked between two plates.
2 Dry the roes well on paper towels. Arrange in a single layer on a large heat-proof plate. Add the milk, butter and a little seasoning.
3 Place the plate over a saucepan of boiling water, cover with a second plate and cook for 10–12 minutes or until the flesh is opaque.
4 Lift from the liquid and serve topped with a dusting of paprika or cayenne. Toasted Corn Bread (see page 222) or Blinis (see page 212) are good accompaniments.

Variation
❋ Put the ingredients into a saucepan, bring the milk to the boil, lower the heat and cook for 8–10 minutes. Serve as above.

Do not freeze

Sautéed Cod's Roe

Cod's roe is most nutritious and can be used in many ways. Most fish counters sell it already cooked, so it simply needs frying, but if you have to buy it uncooked see step 1 below.

Ingredients

Metric (Imperial)	American
450g (1lb) cod's roe	1lb
sea salt and freshly ground white pepper to taste	
50g (2oz) butter	¼ cup
1 tablespoon sunflower or groundnut oil	1¼ tablespoons

Method

1 If the roe is uncooked place it in a steamer with a little seasoning. Cover and cook over boiling water for 10–15 minutes, until the roe loses its translucent appearance.
2 Cool slightly, then remove the outer skin and cut the roe into slices.
3 Heat the butter and oil in a large frying pan (skillet) and heat the slices for 2 minutes. Turn them over and cook for the same time on the second side. Serve hot. Fried or grilled (broiled) mushrooms are a good accompaniment.

Freezing
The uncooked cod's roe can be frozen.

Enjoying Liver

As you will see from the initial menus, calves' or lambs' liver is an essential part of the diet and should be eaten regularly. It should be a most enjoyable meat, full of flavour, moist and tender. Here are a few tips to ensure that you achieve this.

- If you find the flavour slightly too strong for your taste marinate the slices for one person in 3–4 tablespoons of milk before cooking. Leave for 30 minutes, then remove the liver and dry it well on paper towels. The milk, which reduces the strong taste, can be heated with seasoning and chopped herbs, thickened with cornflour and served as a sauce. Note: this step is not suitable for kosher diets.
- Never overcook liver. This does not make it more tender; on the contrary it makes it hard and dry. It cooks extremely quickly, so I never do it in the microwave. Neither do I flour it before cooking. I find this tends to harden the outside; and of course while following the diet you should omit a flour coating in any form of cooking.
- If you are serving other ingredients, such as onions, as an accompaniment to liver, cook them first and keep them warm, *then* cook the liver. Never keep liver waiting on the hot pan, as it will continue to cook; serve it immediately.

As you will see from the following recipes there are many ingredients that blend well with liver. Do try them, for they make a pleasant change. The liver recipes covering the first 14 days of the diet are very simple, as they use just the recommended ingredients. After you have discovered which foods do, and do not, affect your arthritis you can become more adventurous.

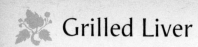

Grilled Liver

Grilling (broiling) is one good way of cooking liver. It is also the way of preparing liver as required by Jewish dietary laws – see under Variations.

Ingredients

METRIC (IMPERIAL)	AMERICAN
2 slices of calves' liver, about 1cm (⅓ inch) thick	2
1 tablespoon butter, melted or olive oil	1¼ tablespoons
tsea salt and freshly ground black pepper to taste	

Method

1 Wash the liver in cold water, then dry thoroughly on paper towels.
2 Preheat the grill (broiler) and spread a piece of foil over the wire grid. Place the liver slices on this, brush with the butter or oil and season lightly.
3 Cook for about 1 minute only, then turn over, brush with the remaining butter or oil and season again. Cook for the same time on the second side; remove immediately and serve at once.

Variations

🌾 The butter or oil can be flavoured with a little ground ginger or grated ginger root or with ground cinnamon or chilli powder.
🌾 Finely grated lemon or orange zest are other good additions (if you are sure these do not affect your arthritis).
🌾 This is also a good method of cooking lambs' and chicken livers.
🌾 Jewish dietary recommendations: grilling (broiling) is the method recommended for preparing all kinds of liver. The slices should first be lightly scored so the blood runs out, laid on foil in a special grill pan, sprinkled with kitchen salt and grilled as above. Butter or oil is not used. It is essential to take this step before cooking the liver in other ways. Always discard the foil.

Do not freeze

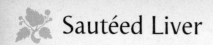# Sautéed Liver

Calves' liver is the ideal choice but as this is more expensive than lambs' liver you may choose to fry that instead. Cut lambs' liver even thinner than recommended for calves' liver. Do not forget chicken livers, as they are equally good when fried. As liver is so important in this initial attack on arthritis do spoil yourself and choose the meat that pleases you most. I have not specified the weight of liver; you can judge this for yourself. Buy two fairly large slices.

Liver is very lean, so you should be fairly generous with the amount of fat used.

Ingredients

SERVES 1

METRIC (IMPERIAL)	AMERICAN
2 slices of calves' liver, about 1cm (⅓ inch) thick	2
sea salt and freshly ground black pepper to taste	
25g (1oz) butter	2 tablespoons
2 teaspoons sunflower oil	2 teaspoons

Method

1 Wash the liver in cold water, dry thoroughly on paper towels and season lightly.
2 Heat the butter and oil in a large frying pan (skillet). Fry the liver for about 1 minute, then turn over and fry for the same time on the second side. Remove immediately and serve at once.

Variations

❋ Lambs' liver and chicken livers may need another ¹/₂–1 minute's cooking on either side to suit the tastes of some people.

❋ *Liver with Mixed Herbs:* add 2 (2¹/₂) tablespoons of mixed coarsely chopped herbs to the butter and oil before frying the liver. A good selection would be sage, chervil or parsley, chives and tarragon. If you want to use one herb only sage leaves are a very good choice.

❋ *Gravy to serve with liver:* the ideal time to make this is when the liver is cooked on one side only. Have ready a teaspoon of cornflour (cornstarch) mixed with 175ml (6fl oz/³/₄ cup) of chicken or vegetable stock (bouillon). Pour over the liver in the frying pan, turn the meat over and stir briskly as the gravy thickens and the liver finishes cooking. You could also add 1 or 2 teaspoons of prepared English or Dijon mustard to the pan. Instead of all stock you could use half stock and half single (light) cream.

❋ *Liver with Avocado:* halve, stone and peel a small avocado, then cut the flesh into neat slices. Sprinkle these with a little cider vinegar or rice vinegar (or lemon juice if you are happy with citrus fruit). Fry briefly in the butter and oil, then move to one side of the pan and fry the liver.

❋ *Liver with Kiwi Fruit:* wash and dry the liver as in step 1, place on a plate and cover with thin slices of peeled kiwi fruit. Leave for an hour, then fry the fruit and liver together. The acidity of kiwi fruit flavours and tenderizes liver. It is particularly good with chicken livers or lambs' liver.

❋ *Liver and Onions:* if preparing this dish for several people it is almost easier to work with two frying pans. If using one frying pan for one person this is the method to use. Heat a good tablespoon of oil in a pan and fry 1 medium to large thinly sliced onion – the slices should be pulled apart to form rings. Cook these fairly slowly, adding a little seasoning as you do so. To give a slightly caramelized taste to the onion stir in a teaspoon of honey or sugar. When the onions are tender put on to a well-heated dish and keep hot in the oven, or move to one side of the frying pan while frying the liver.

Do not freeze

Chicken Liver Risotto

This is one of the best-known Italian rice dishes. The classic name is
Risotto alla Finanziera. To avoid overcooking the livers do not add them
at the beginning of the cooking period. Risotto (medium grain) rice is
easily obtainable; the most common one is called arborio. It may sound
troublesome to add the hot liquid gradually but this is essential to
achieve the desired moist texture. If you have difficulty finding fresh
chicken livers buy frozen ones; defrost and dry them well.

You will find cooked rice is an excellent accompaniment to many
main dishes instead of potatoes, which are one of the nightshade vegetables you have to avoid during the initial steps of the diet. Choose organic
brown rice whenever possible.

Ingredients   SERVES 4

METRIC (IMPERIAL)	AMERICAN
2 tablespoons olive oil	2½ tablespoons
1 medium onion, finely chopped	1
1 or 2 garlic cloves, finely chopped	1 or 2
350g (12oz) arborio or other risotto rice	good 1½ cups
225g (8oz) chicken livers	good 1 cup
1.2 litres (2 pints) chicken stock (bouillon), (see page 98)	5 cups
sea salt and freshly ground black pepper to taste	
100g (3½ oz) small button mushrooms, optional	1 cup
25g (1oz) butter	2 tablespoons

To garnish
chopped tarragon leaves

Method

1   Heat the oil in a large saucepan, add the onion and cook gently for 5
    minutes, then stir in the garlic and cook for a further 2 minutes.

2   Add the rice and turn in the oil mixture, so all the grains become coated. Remove any gristle from the livers and dice them neatly.

3   Meanwhile, heat the stock in another saucepan. Add just enough of the hot stock to moisten the rice mixture, and when this has been absorbed add a little more. Stir in salt and pepper to taste.

4   Continue adding hot stock until the rice is beginning to soften, then stir in the liver, and the mushrooms if using. Watch the pan carefully and as soon as the rice absorbs the hot liquid add more. Stop when the rice is just tender; the finished dish should still be moist.

5   Check the seasoning and stir in the butter. Top with the tarragon and serve.

Variations

🌸 Although never included in the classic recipe you can stir in 3 (3¾) tablespoons raisins just before the rice is cooked. The sweetness of the dried fruit balances the flavour well.

🌸 When you can include most cheeses in your diet top the dish with grated Parmesan and serve it as an accompaniment.

🌸 Instead of fresh mushrooms soak 1 (1¼) tablespoons porcini (dried mushrooms) in a little hot water as instructed on the packet, then add to the other ingredients.

🌸 To give a touch of luxury to the risotto add a few drops of truffle oil to the stock.

🌸 There are many other foods you can use instead of chicken livers but during the vital first days of the diet the livers are important. Try the following:

Chickpea (garbanzo bean) and Liver Risotto: add 175g (6oz) or 1 good cup cooked chickpeas to the risotto at step 4 after putting in the liver and mushrooms. (Chickpeas have an excellent flavour and high protein value, so should be served as often as possible.)

Mushroom Risotto: use about 450g (1lb) diced mixed mushrooms, including as many wild varieties as possible.

Freezing

Cook to the end of step 4. Cool and freeze.

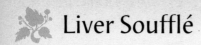

Liver Soufflé

This is an excellent way to introduce liver to anyone who is not over-fond of the flavour. It gets them accustomed to the taste.

Ingredients

SERVES 2 AS A MAIN COURSE

METRIC (IMPERIAL)	AMERICAN
1 tablespoon sunflower oil	1¼ tablespoons
175g (6oz) button mushrooms, sliced	1 cup
150g (5oz) calves' or lambs' liver, minced (ground) or very finely chopped	good ½ cup
25g (1oz) butter or margarine	2 tablespoons
15g (½oz) cornflour (cornstarch)	1 tablespoon
150ml (5fl oz) milk or chicken stock (bouillon)	⅔ cup
3 large eggs	3
1 egg white	1
sea salt and freshly ground black pepper to taste	

Method

1 Lightly grease a 15–18cm (6–7 inch) soufflé dish. Heat the oil in a frying pan (skillet), add the mushrooms and cook for 3 minutes. Spoon about three-quarters into the base of the soufflé dish. Mix the remaining mushrooms with the uncooked liver.

2 Preheat the oven to 190°C/375°F/Gas Mark 5 or 180°C for a fan (convection) oven.

3 Heat the butter or margarine in a large saucepan, stir in the cornflour and cook gently for 1 minute. Gradually add the milk or stock. Bring to the boil, then lower the heat and stir until the sauce thickens.

4 Remove the saucepan from the heat and stir in the mushroom and liver mixture. Separate the eggs and put the 3 whites into a bowl with the extra egg white.

5 Beat the yolks, then stir into the ingredients in the saucepan. Add a little seasoning.

6 Whisk the whites until they stand in soft peaks. Take a few spoonfuls and beat into the liver mixture to give a softer consistency. Gently fold in the remainder. Taste and adjust the seasoning.

7 Spoon into the prepared soufflé dish and bake for 30–35 minutes or until well-risen. Serve at once with a mixed salad.

Do not freeze

Country Lambs' Kidneys

*Lamb and veal kidneys are important foods in this diet. As they are
tender meats they are quick to prepare and cook. I have suggested using
spring onions (scallions) in this recipe as they look attractive and, like
the kidneys, are quick to cook. Alternatively, you could use very small
shallots, pickling (pearl) onions or thinly sliced mild onions.*

Ingredients   SERVES 4

METRIC (IMPERIAL)	AMERICAN
450g (1lb) lambs' kidneys	1lb
1 tablespoon cornflour (cornstarch)	1¼ tablespoons
sea salt and freshly ground black pepper to taste	
25g (1oz) butter	2 tablespoons
2 tablespoons sunflower or groundnut oil	2½ tablespoons
225g (8oz) plump spring onions (scallions) (trimmed weight)	½lb
225g (8oz) small button mushrooms	½lb
300ml (10fl oz) plus extra if required meat or chicken stock (bouillon) (see pages 98–99)	1¼ cups plus extra if required

To garnish
watercress sprigs

Method

1 Skin the kidneys and cut each one in half; remove any gristle and excess fat. Mix the cornflour with a little salt and pepper and use to coat the kidneys.

2 Heat the butter and half the oil in a saucepan. Add the kidneys and cook steadily, turning them around several times, for 5 minutes. Remove from the pan on to a plate.

3 Check the amount of fat left in the saucepan; if little is left add the remaining oil, heat and add the onions. Cook for about 5 minutes, turning once or twice, until they are slightly golden.

4 Return the kidneys to the pan with the mushrooms and stock. Bring the liquid to the boil, check the seasoning, then cover the pan and simmer for 10–15 minutes or until all the ingredients are tender. Check during the cooking time to see there is sufficient liquid; if not add more stock.

5 Garnish and serve with cooked brown rice and mixed vegetables.

Variation

❀ *Sautéed Kidneys:* skin then slice lambs' kidneys or veal kidney. Do not coat in cornflour, just season lightly. Fry steadily in hot butter and oil, or all oil, until tender.

Freezing

Proceed to the end of step 4, cool and freeze.

Creamed Sweetbreads

Sweetbreads are another valuable food to include in your arthritis diet. Veal sweetbreads are not readily available but the smaller lambs' sweetbreads are very good. You may have to purchase them frozen, in which case defrost and dry well before using. Classic recipes suggest that sweetbreads are first pressed under a weight, then sliced before using, but this rather laborious step is not necessary.

Soya milk could be used in the sauce; it gives an interesting change of flavour.

Ingredients
SERVES 4

METRIC (IMPERIAL)	AMERICAN
550g (1¼lb) sweetbreads	1¼lb
1–2 medium onions, sliced	1–2
2 medium carrots, sliced	2
small bunch parsley	small bunch
sea salt and freshly ground white pepper to taste	

For the sauce

25g (1oz) butter	2 tablespoons
15g (½oz) cornflour (cornstarch)	2 tablespoons
150ml (5fl oz) milk	⅔ cup
150ml (5fl oz) sweetbread stock (bouillon), (see method)	⅔ cup
150ml (5fl oz) single (light) cream or extra milk	⅔ cup
2 tablespoons chopped parsley or other herbs	2½ tablespoons

Method

1 Wash the sweetbreads in cold water, then put into a saucepan, cover with water and bring to the boil. Strain immediately, discarding the water. This is known as blanching, a process which whitens the meat.

2 Return the sweetbreads to the pan with the onion(s), carrots, parsley and enough water to cover. Add a little seasoning. Simmer steadily for about 20 minutes for lambs' sweetbreads or up to 30 minutes for veal sweetbreads.

3 Strain and retain 150ml (5fl oz) or $\frac{2}{3}$ cup of the stock. Remove the skin and any gristle from the sweetbreads. Larger sweetbreads should be cut into neat dice.

4 Heat the butter in a saucepan. Mix the cornflour with the milk and add to the pan with the stock. Stir as the liquid comes to the boil and thickens, then add the cream or extra milk and the diced sweetbreads. Heat well, then stir in half the parsley and any seasoning required. Top with the remaining parsley and serve with mixed vegetables.

Do not freeze

Sweet and Sour Lambs' Hearts

Hearts are a very good alternative to liver, and lambs' hearts are the most tender. The meat is very lean, so it fits perfectly into a low-fat diet.

Ingredients

METRIC (IMPERIAL)	AMERICAN
8 small lambs' hearts	8
sea salt and freshly ground black pepper to taste	
1 tablespoon cornflour (cornstarch)	1¼ tablespoons
2 tablespoons sunflower oil	2½ tablespoons
2 medium onions, finely chopped	2
150ml (5fl oz) lamb stock (bouillon) (see page 99)	⅔ cup
150ml (5fl oz) apple juice	⅔ cup
3 teaspoons honey	3 teaspoons
1 tablespoon balsamic or other vinegar	1¼ tablespoons
2 dessert apples, cored, peeled and cut into rings	2
2 tablespoons raisins	2½ tablespoons

To garnish
watercress

Method

1   Preheat the oven to 160°C/325°F/Gas Mark 3 or 150°C for a fan (convection) oven.
2   Skin the hearts, remove any gristle and fat, then cut the meat into fingers about 2cm (³/₄ inch) wide. Mix a little seasoning with the cornflour and use to coat the meat.
3   Heat half the oil in a frying pan (skillet), add the onions and sauté for 3 minutes only; spoon into a casserole.
4   Add the remaining oil to the pan, heat again, then stir in the strips of heart. Cook gently for 5 minutes, turning over halfway through the cooking time. Spoon into the casserole.
5   Pour the stock and apple juice into the pan. Stir well to absorb all the meat juices, then stir in the honey and vinegar and bring the mixture just to boiling point. Pour over the meat. Cover and cook for 1 hour.
6   Add the apple rings and the raisins, taste the liquid and add more seasoning if required. Cover again and cook for a further 30 minutes. Garnish and serve. Sweet potatoes, baked in their skins and cooked red cabbage are good accompaniments.

Freezing
The dish is better if frozen without the apples. These become over-soft, so add them when reheating.

Curried Tripe

The food value of tripe has been appreciated since Roman times but it is a variety meat that has become somewhat unfashionable. This recipe gives it an up-to-the-minute taste.

Most tripe on sale today has been dressed – prepared – by the butcher so the cooking time is considerably reduced. If by chance you are sold undressed tripe simmer it slowly in water for at least 1 hour, then drain and proceed as below.

Ingredients

SERVES 4

METRIC (IMPERIAL)	AMERICAN
675g (1½lb) tripe, cut into 7.5cm (3 inch) squares	1½lb
1 tablespoon sunflower oil	1¼ tablespoons
25g (1oz) butter	2 tablespoons
2 medium onions, thinly sliced	2
2 garlic cloves, chopped	2
1–2 teaspoons grated root ginger	1–2 teaspoons
½ teaspoon turmeric	½ teaspoon
¼ teaspoon, or to taste cayenne pepper°	¼ teaspoon, or to taste
¼ teaspoon, or to taste chilli powder°	¼ teaspoon, or to taste
1 teaspoon, or to taste ground coriander	1 teaspoon, or to taste
¼ teaspoon ground cumin	¼ teaspoon
300ml (10fl oz), or as required chicken stock (bouillon) or water (see page 98)	1¼ cups, or as required
sea salt to taste	
few drops balsamic or other vinegar to taste	

To garnish
sliced banana and diced pineapple

Method

1 Put the tripe into a saucepan with water to cover, bring to the boil, then strain and discard the liquid. This is known as blanching the tripe and it improves both colour and taste. Do this even if you have had to boil the tripe first.

2 Heat the oil and butter in a saucepan, add the onions and cook gently for 5 minutes. Add the garlic, ginger and all the spices. Stir over a low heat for 2–3 minutes.

3 Pour in the stock or water and bring to simmering point. Add the tripe with salt to taste and the vinegar.

4 Cover the pan and simmer gently for 15 minutes or until the tripe is tender. Check during this period and add a little more stock if required. Garnish and serve with a selection of diced, lightly cooked root vegetables and a green salad.

Freezing
Cook to the end of step 4 but omit the garnish. Add this when reheating the defrosted curry.

*The combination of these two hot spices may be too strong for some people so use them sparingly until you are happy with the result

Steak with Roquefort

This is a simple and very delicious dish using prime beef. When you feel you have gained good control over your arthritis you will want to proceed to more familiar foods, such as various meats and vegetarian dishes. At first it is wise to keep to fairly simple recipes so you can assess their effect easily.

In the case of this recipe do not serve it with an accompaniment of lots of nightshade foods, such as red and green (bell) peppers, tomatoes and potatoes, unless you have proved quite conclusively that these do not adversely affect your arthritis.

I have suggested Roquefort cheese as the topping for the steaks, as this is one of the cheeses you may well have eaten during the initial days of the diet and found it suits you well. Later on you can try other cheeses.

Ingredients

Serves 4

Metric (Imperial)	**American**
50g (2oz) butter	¼ cup
100g (3½oz) Roquefort cheese, crumbled	½ cup
1 tablespoon finely chopped watercress leaves or parsley	1¼ tablespoons
4 fillet or rump steaks	4
sea salt and freshly ground black pepper to taste	

To garnish
cooked mushrooms
watercress or parsley

Method

1 Cream half the butter with the cheese and watercress or parsley.

2 Melt the remaining butter. Preheat the grill (broiler) and place a piece of foil over the grid of the grill pan. Brush this with a little of the melted butter.

3 Put the steaks on the foil, brush with butter and season to taste. Cook for 1–2 minutes only, then turn and brush with the rest of the butter. Cook for a further 2–6 minutes, depending upon how well done you like your steak.

4 Top the steaks with the Roquefort mixture about 2 minutes before the end of the cooking time, so the cheese just starts to melt. Garnish and serve.

Variations

✻ Fillets of lamb (slices from the leg); or veal, chicken or turkey escalopes are excellent served the same way.

Do not freeze

Caribbean Lamb

When moving from the initial diet do try this dish, which gives lamb a great deal of flavour. The combination of chilli powder and refreshing pineapple is a very pleasant one. If you find that red and green (bell) peppers and chilli peppers do not affect your arthritis adversely then they can be included for extra taste and texture (see under Variations).

Add the chilli powder gradually as different makes vary in strength.

Ingredients

SERVES 4

METRIC (IMPERIAL)	AMERICAN
1 tablespoon sunflower or groundnut oil	1¼ tablespoons
1 large onion, finely chopped	1
1 or 2 garlic cloves, finely chopped	1 or 2
½–1 teaspoon chilli powder	½–1 teaspoon
8 lamb cutlets	8
150ml (5fl oz) pineapple juice	⅔ cup
2–3 fresh pineapple slices	2–3
sea salt to taste	

To garnish
diced seasonal vegetables

Method

1 Heat the oil in a large frying pan (skillet), add the onion and cook gently for 5 minutes, then add the garlic and chilli powder. Stir over a low heat for 1 minute to bring out the flavour of the chilli.

2 Add the cutlets and turn around in the pan so they become coated with the chilli mixture, then sauté for 2 minutes on each side. Pour in the pineapple juice. Lower the heat and cook gently for 5 minutes or until the meat is almost cooked to your personal taste.

3 Meanwhile, cut away the peel from the pineapple and remove the centre hard core; dice the fruit neatly. Add to the pan and heat for 1–2 minutes. Garnish and serve.

Variations

* Use 4 large lamb chops instead of the cutlets. Remove any surplus fat from these before cooking.

* If you can eat peppers then use 1 deseeded and finely chopped chilli pepper instead of chilli powder and add 4 (5) tablespoons of diced red and green peppers just before the pineapple.

* Thin slices of lean, tender pork can be used instead of lamb cutlets.

Do not freeze

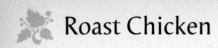

Roast Chicken

Roast chicken is allowed in the first few days of the diet, and is a good alternative to liver and fish. Ordinary meats are not recommended while you are following the first very important days of the diet. You can, however, serve turkey or game birds instead of chicken. If you can, use organically-reared poultry and game birds – these are now much more readily available.

Ingredients

METRIC (IMPERIAL)	AMERICAN
1 young roasting chicken – about 2kg (4½lb) in weight when trussed	1
2 tablespoons butter, softened or olive oil	2½ tablespoons
sea salt and freshly ground black pepper to taste	
flavourings – see opposite	

Method

1   Wash the chicken well in cold water, dry very thoroughly and put into a roasting tin (pan).

2   Good-quality birds can be roasted at a high temperature, so preheat the oven to 220°C/425°F/Gas Mark 7 or 210°C for a fan (convection) oven.

3   Brush the bird with the butter or olive oil, paying special attention to the breast. Season lightly.

4   Roast for about 1½ hours. You can baste the chicken with a little more butter or oil halfway through the cooking time. If cooking birds of a different weight, allow 15 minutes per 450g (1lb) and 15 minutes extra.

5   Check carefully before serving. Pierce the bird where the leg joins the body and note the colour of the juice that flows. If it is at all pink then the bird needs a little longer cooking. When it is done the liquid will be clear.

6   Cover the bird with foil and leave to stand for 10 minutes before carving.

Variations

❋ Turkey, guinea fowl and game birds need about the same cooking time. (See Quail recipe on page 156.)

❋ With larger chickens or turkeys cook for half the time with the breast side downwards, then turn over to complete cooking. This helps to keep the breast moist.

❋ If you lay foil over the bird while roasting you need to allow another 5–10 minutes' cooking time

❋ If you prefer slower roasting, preheat the oven to 180°C/350°F/Gas Mark 4 or 170°C for a fan (convection) oven. Allow 25 minutes per 450g (1lb) and 25 minutes extra.

Flavourings

❋ Remember that you must avoid stuffings based on bread, sausages and bacon during the initial diet, and also the juice from citrus fruits.

❋ It is not recommended that moist mixtures, such as the Almond Relish on page 168, are put in the cavity of the bird. Put them under the skin at the neck end or between the skin and the breast meat.

❋ One or two peeled, whole garlic cloves or a peeled onion can be put into the body of the bird to give additional flavouring; or you could put a small bunch of mixed herbs such as parsley, chives, rosemary and thyme in the bird.

❋ The melted butter or oil used to brush over the bird can be flavoured with crushed garlic, grated root ginger, or chopped herbs such as thyme, tarragon or rosemary. Alternatively, mix a little sesame oil with the butter or olive oil and sprinkle sesame seeds over the bird when nearly cooked.

❋ If you find citrus fruit does not affect your arthritis then one of the best ways of flavouring chicken is with lemon. Put a halved lemon inside the bird and sprinkle the uncooked flesh with lemon juice before brushing with butter or oil.

Do not freeze

Turkey in Almond Sauce

This recipe uses turkey fillets (tender slices of breast meat), which are readily available. Check carefully to ensure you are buying fillets from organic turkey. The addition of a generous amount of coriander (cilantro) is important as it adds both flavour and colour. The sauce keeps the turkey flesh moist. If you dislike coriander use tarragon instead.

Ingredients

SERVES 4

METRIC (IMPERIAL)	AMERICAN
2 tablespoons sunflower oil	2½ tablespoons
4 turkey fillets	4
2 small onions, finely chopped	2
1 garlic clove, finely chopped	1
50g (2oz) blanched almonds, chopped	½ cup
sea salt and freshly ground black pepper to taste	
150ml (5fl oz) crème fraîche	⅔ cup
4 tablespoons chicken stock (bouillon) (see page 98)	5 tablespoons
1½ tablespoons chopped coriander (cilantro)	1¾ tablespoons

To garnish
paprika
coriander (cilantro) leaves

Method

1 Heat the oil in a large frying pan (skillet), add the turkey fillets and cook fairly quickly until just golden brown on both sides. Remove from the pan with a perforated spoon or fish slice.

2 Add the onions to the pan and heat steadily for 4 minutes, then add the garlic and almonds and stir over a low heat until the almonds turn pale golden. The onions and garlic can be allowed to colour slightly too, but take care they do not burn.

3 Return the turkey to the pan and add seasoning. Stir in the crème fraîche and stock and simmer gently, stirring from time to time, for about 10 minutes or until the turkey is tender. Stir the coriander into the sauce just before serving. Top with a good dusting of paprika and coriander leaves. Serve with cooked brown rice and broccoli.

Variations

* Chicken breast portions can be cooked in the same way.
* Yoghurt or fromage frais could be used instead of crème fraîche.

Do not freeze

Quail with Blueberry Sauce

These small game birds are available throughout the year, and many supermarkets sell them ready boned. They are surprisingly meaty, so while I suggest allowing two per person, you may find one is enough for those with small appetites. A classic way of cooking quail is to wrap them in vine leaves. These prevent the delicate flesh from drying out, and are eaten along with the birds. Since these are not easy to obtain I often use tender leaves from a cabbage heart instead.

Ingredients

SERVES 4

METRIC (IMPERIAL)	AMERICAN
16–24 vine leaves or about 8 young cabbage leaves	16–24
sea salt and freshly ground black pepper to taste	
40g (1½oz) butter	3 tablespoons
8 quail	8
For the sauce	
150ml (5fl oz) water	⅔ cup
1 tablespoon honey	1¼ tablespoons
225g (8oz) blueberries	1¾ cups

Method

1 Preheat the oven to 200°C/400°F/Gas Mark 6 or 190°C for a fan (convection) oven.

2 If using vine leaves wash and drain them well; if young they do not need heating but if older treat as cabbage. To heat the leaves, put a small amount of water into a saucepan, season lightly and bring to the boil. Add the leaves and boil for 1 minute only, then drain.

3 Place the leaves on a work surface. Spread the butter over the quail and season. Put each bird on enough leaves to enclose it completely when wrapped round.

4 Lift the parcels into a roasting tin (pan) or large ovenproof dish. Cover with foil or a lid and cook for 25–30 minutes.

5 To make the sauce, put the water and honey into a saucepan or bowl in the microwave. Bring to boiling point then add the blueberries and cook gently until tender.

6 Serve the quail parcels with the sauce poured around them. Roasted parsnips and/or sweet potatoes are excellent accompaniments; as is a crisp green salad.

Variation

🌿 Pheasant or guinea fowl: either of these birds can be cooked the same way. Spread the birds with Creamy Liver Pâté (see page 92) instead of butter.

Do not freeze

Salmis of Pheasant

This is a classic recipe that I have adjusted to avoid the use of flour, which contains wheat. Wheat flour is normally used to thicken the sauce, but here I have used cornflour (cornstarch), which comes from maize. Use cornflour for thickening gravies and other sauces too. Remember it has twice the thickening ability of ordinary flour, so where a standard recipe states 25g (1oz /¼ cup) of flour use half that amount of cornflour. This is an ideal dish to choose when entertaining as the pheasant looks pleasantly brown and there is no last-minute carving to be done.

Ingredients   SERVES 4–6

METRIC (IMPERIAL)	AMERICAN
2 large pheasants, lightly roasted (see page 156)	2 large
900ml (1½ pints) water	3¾ cups
sea salt and freshly ground black pepper to taste	
1 small bunch mixed herbs – parsley, thyme, rosemary and marjoram	1 small bunch
2 fresh bay leaves	2
3 medium shallots, roughly chopped	3
3 medium carrots, roughly chopped	3
100g (3½oz) button mushrooms	1 cup
½ teaspoon turmeric	½ teaspoon
½ teaspoon grated nutmeg	½ teaspoon
25g (1oz) cornflour	¼ cup
3 tablespoons sherry or port (not while on the strict diet) or water	3¾ tablespoons

To garnish

2 fresh pineapple rings	2

Method

1 Cut away the leg joints from the birds and halve them. Cut away the breast joints, making sure they are kept intact. If very large and plump these too can be halved.

2 Break the carcass into small pieces and place in a saucepan with the water and a little seasoning. Bring to the boil, then cover the pan and lower the heat.

3 Simmer for 45 minutes, then strain the liquid and return it to the pan.

4 Tie the herbs with cotton, so they can be removed easily, and put into the stock with the bay leaves, shallots, carrots, mushrooms, turmeric and nutmeg.

5 Simmer for 30 minutes; then remove the bunch of herbs and the bay leaves. Mix the cornflour with the sherry, port or water, add to the hot liquid and stir to make a smooth, slightly thickened sauce.

6 Spoon the sauce and vegetables into a liquidizer or food processor and process to a thin, smooth purée. Taste and adjust the seasoning.

7 Preheat the oven to 170°C/325°F/Gas Mark 3 or 150°C for a fan (convection) oven.

8 Pour the sauce into a casserole and lay the pheasant joints in it. Cover and cook for 35–40 minutes. Do not overcook.

9 Cut away the skin and hard core from the pineapple rings. Dice the flesh and use to garnish the Salmis. Serve with a selection of vegetables. Mashed celeriac is a particularly good accompaniment.

Variation

🌿 Any game birds can be served in the same way.

Freezing

This particular dish is better not frozen.

Cucumber Sauce

Do not overlook the value of cucumbers to add flavour and interest to salads and other dishes. Strips of cucumber are also excellent in stir-fries. While you are avoiding nightshade foods, such as tomatoes, sweet (bell) peppers and chilli peppers, you will find these cucumber sauces excellent alternatives with meat such as lamb or veal, or with chicken or fish.

Ingredients

SERVES 4

METRIC (IMPERIAL)	AMERICAN
115g (4oz) small cucumber (peeled weight)	1 cup
25g (1oz) butter	2 tablespoons
15g (½oz) cornflour (cornstarch)	2 tablespoons
300ml (10fl oz) milk	1¼ cups
2 teaspoons or to taste apple, cider or rice vinegar	2 teaspoons or to taste
sea salt and freshly ground white pepper to taste	
herbs, see step 4 to taste	

Method

1   Dice the cucumber, then sieve or liquidize to make a purée.
2   Heat the butter in a saucepan, stir in the cornflour and continue stirring over a low heat for 1–2 minutes. Gradually stir in the milk, then bring the sauce to the boil and whisk or stir briskly until thickened. Stir in the cucumber purée.
3   Lower the heat and simmer gently for 5 minutes, then remove from the heat and whisk in the vinegar.
4   Add a little salt and pepper, then the chopped herbs. Choose mint if serving the sauce with lamb; tarragon or rosemary with chicken; fennel or dill leaves with fish. (Parsley and basil are other herbs that blend well with cucumber.) Heat gently, without boiling, then serve.

Variations

❋ Instead of making the sauce simply mix the cucumber purée, or peeled and coarsely grated cucumber, with 250ml (8fl oz/1 cup) of thick yoghurt. Add the vinegar, seasoning and herbs as in the recipe. Serve cold.

❋ *Cucumber Coulis:* peel and coarsely grate 1 small or ½ large cucumber. Mix with 1 (1¼) tablespoons apple, cider or rice vinegar, seasoning and herbs to taste.

Freezing

Neither version of the sauce freezes well, though the coulis can be frozen. It is better to add the herbs after defrosting.

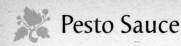

Pesto Sauce

This is a classic sauce to serve with pasta. If you are avoiding wheat products while on the Eat to Beat Arthritis Diet you can still enjoy this sauce with gluten-free pasta, or use it to add extra flavour to fish and a variety of cooked vegetables. If you find that wheat does not adversely affect your arthritis, you can enjoy this sauce with every kind of pasta. Make the sauce with a mixture of herbs or just basil leaves.

Ingredients   SERVES 4

METRIC (IMPERIAL)	AMERICAN
about 8 flat parsley leaves, coarsely shredded	about 8
2 small sprigs marjoram or oregano	2 small sprigs
about 20 basil leaves	about 20
2 garlic cloves	2
75g (scant 3oz) Parmesan cheese, grated	good ½ cup
5 tablespoons extra virgin olive oil	6¼ tablespoons
100g (3½oz) pine (pignolia) nuts	1 cup
sea salt and freshly ground black pepper to taste	

Method

1 Put all the ingredients into a liquidizer or food processor and process to a thick purée. Serve cold.

Variations
* Often 1–2 tablespoons of melted butter are liquidized with the other ingredients to give greater richness to the sauce.
* You can add a second cheese. Pecorino (romano) is an Italian choice, but 2–3 tablespoons of goat's cheese could be used while on the diet.
* Use blanched almonds instead of pine nuts.

Do not freeze

Vinaigrette Dressing

This is the basic dressing for most salads though it can be varied in many ways. Virgin olive oil, which comes from the first pressing of the olives, is the classic choice for a good salad dressing but there will be occasions when you prefer to use other oils. If you are anxious to keep your fat intake low, look for light olive oil. Organic olive and other oils are also obtainable.

Wine vinegar was traditionally mixed with the oil but today there are many other types on the market, and these add individual touches to the dressing. Well-matured balsamic vinegar, though very expensive, can be added in very small quantities to give a delicious sweetness. If you find that citrus fruits do not affect your arthritis adversely you can substitute lemon or lime juice for vinegar.

Ingredients

SERVES 4

METRIC (IMPERIAL)	AMERICAN
1 teaspoon Dijon mustard	1 teaspoon
150ml (5fl oz) virgin olive oil	⅔ cup
4 tablespoons red or white wine vinegar	5 tablespoons
sea salt and freshly ground black pepper to taste	
1 teaspoon sugar or honey	1 teaspoon

Method

1 Put all the ingredients into a bowl or screw-topped jar and whisk or shake briskly. A larger quantity could be mixed together in a liquidizer (blender).

2 Use as required. Any dressing left over can be stored in a covered container for several days in a cool place.

Variations

❋ For a lighter dressing use half olive and half sunflower or other oil. To change the flavour use 2–3 teaspoons sesame seed oil and omit this amount of olive oil. Walnut or other nut oils can be used in the same way.

❋ Substitute 1 tablespoon balsamic vinegar for the same amount of wine vinegar. Do not use more than this as the flavour would be too strong for most salads. You can change the proportions of oil and vinegar according to personal taste.

❋ Add crushed garlic cloves and chopped mixed herbs; or crushed root ginger, galangal or finely chopped lemon grass to the dressing.

❋ Add spices such as chilli powder or cayenne pepper to give a hotter dressing

❋ If you are able to eat nightshade vegetables, add finely diced sun-dried tomatoes, sweet (bell) peppers or hot chilli peppers.

Do not freeze

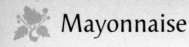

Mayonnaise

While you are avoiding as many prepared foods as possible it is advisable to make your own mayonnaise. This is not difficult, particularly if you use a liquidizer or food processor.

Bring the eggs out of the refrigerator about 1 hour before making the sauce as this helps to ensure a smooth mayonnaise.

Ingredients

SERVES 4–6

METRIC (IMPERIAL)	AMERICAN
2 yolks, from large eggs	2
1 teaspoon Dijon mustard	1 teaspoon
sea salt and freshly ground white pepper to taste	
up to 300ml (10fl oz) extra virgin olive oil*	up to 1¼ cups
3 teaspoons white wine or rice vinegar	3 teaspoons
1 tablespoon very hot water, optional	1¼ tablespoons

*This amount of oil is the maximum most people would like, so you can reduce it to give a less oily dressing. The choice of oils can be varied, see under Vinaigrette Dressing, page 164

Method

1 Put the egg yolks into a bowl, add the mustard and seasoning and stir well. Gradually add the oil. The best way to do this is to hold the container in one hand and trickle the oil slowly on to the yolks, while stirring or whisking briskly with the other hand. Stop immediately if there is the slightest sign of the sauce curdling (separating). If this happens, whisk very hard indeed.

2 If the sauce has already curdled, break a third egg yolk into a second bowl and gradually whisk in the curdled sauce. When sufficient oil for your taste has been absorbed and the sauce has thickened, stir in the vinegar.

3 If the mayonnaise is very thick and you would prefer a lighter sauce, whisk in the hot water.

Variations

❋ Using a liquidizer or food processsor: when making mayonnaise in this way you can use whole eggs, rather than just the yolks. This produces a lighter sauce. Put the whole eggs or egg yolks into the goblet or bowl, add the seasonings and, *with the motor running,* slowly pour in the oil. When the sauce has thickened add the vinegar, and hot water if using this.

❋ *Hard-boiled (Hard-cooked) Egg Mayonnaise:* if you prefer not to use uncooked eggs substitute the yolks of 2 hard-boiled eggs for the raw egg yolks.

Do not freeze

Almond Relish

*This relish is included in the first week's diet as an accompaniment to
chicken. It is delicious with most poultry, so suggestions for varying the
flavour are given. Lemon juice would normally be used in such a recipe
but in this version the wonderful herb lemon balm is used, along with
lemon grass.*

Ingredients

Metric (Imperial)	American
2 tablespoons olive oil	2½ tablespoons
1 medium onion, finely chopped	1
50g (2oz) raisins	⅓ cup
1 large barely ripe dessert pear, peeled and finely diced	1 large
115g (4oz) tenderized (ready to eat) dried apricots, finely chopped	⅔ cup
115g (4oz) whole or blanched almonds, chopped	1 cup
50g (2oz) ground almonds	½ cup
1 lemon grass stalk, finely chopped	1
1 tablespoon finely chopped lemon balm or ½ tablespoon dried lemon balm	1¼ tablespoons
sea salt and freshly ground black pepper to taste	

Method

1 Heat the oil in a saucepan and cook the onion for 5 minutes; remove from the heat. Stir in the remaining ingredients and season.
2 Some of the stuffing can be inserted under the skin at the neck end of the bird and the remainder cooked in a separate dish, which should be covered.
3 Cook for 40 minutes in a preheated oven set to 190°C/375°F/Gas Mark 5 or 180°C for a fan (convection) oven.

Variations

* If you find that citrus fruit does not affect your arthritis substitute 1–1¼ (1¼–1½) tablespoons of lemon juice for the lemon grass and lemon balm.
* This stuffing is equally good with turkey or guinea fowl. You could use walnuts instead of almonds.
* With duck or goose: substitute a large apple for the pear. Use a cooking (baking) apple to give a sharper flavour and a dessert apple for a sweeter taste.

Do not freeze

Herbed Polenta

Polenta is made from maize flour and is very filling, so makes an ideal alternative to wheat products and potatoes. Authentic polenta needs to be cooked very slowly and stirred constantly, but this recipe is based on the quick-cooking variety. It is possible to buy ready-cooked polenta but wiser to avoid this while on the strict diet. If you wish to make the dish with authentic polenta see Variations below.

Ingredients

SERVES 4

METRIC (IMPERIAL)	**AMERICAN**
900ml (1½ pints) water	3¾ cups
1 teaspoon sea salt	1 teaspoon
225g (8oz) instant polenta	1½ cups
good pinch freshly ground black pepper	good pinch
2 tablespoons finely chopped parsley	2½ tablespoons
1 tablespoon finely snipped chives	1¼ tablespoons
1 tablespoon olive oil	1¼ tablespoons
For frying	
3 tablespoons olive oil	3¾ tablespoons

Method

1 Pour the water into a saucepan and bring to the boil. Add the salt, then slowly and steadily pour in the polenta.

2 Lower the heat, add the pepper and herbs and continue stirring until thickened; this takes about 4 minutes.

3 Brush a shallow dish or tin with the oil and spoon the polenta in to it, spreading evenly to give a depth of about 2.5cm (1 inch). Leave until cool.

4 Dip a sharp knife into boiling water and cut the polenta into fingers. You could use a pastry cutter instead to give more interesting shapes.

5 Heat the olive oil in a frying pan (skillet) and fry the polenta on either side until golden brown. Serve hot with cooked fish, liver, poultry or game.

Variations

If using authentic polenta, let it run through your fingers like sand into the boiling salted water. Cook steadily, stirring all the time, for about 45 minutes. Add the pepper and herbs as described above.

Freezing

Polenta freezes well. Open-freeze, then pack.

Savoury Omelettes

An omelette is a quick and easy dish for any meal of the day. I have suggested serving them as a breakfast dish. One filling – of prawns (shrimp) – may be unusual for breakfast but it ensures that you have fish on that particular day.

Ingredients

METRIC (IMPERIAL)	AMERICAN
2 or 3 large eggs	2 or 3
1 tablespoon water, optional	1¼ tablespoons
sea salt and freshly ground black pepper to taste	
25g (1oz) butter	2 tablespoons
few drops olive or sunflower oil, optional	few drops

Method

1 Lightly beat the eggs with a fork; do not whisk hard, as that aerates the mixture too much and makes it become slightly drier in cooking. Add the water if desired; this gives a lighter texture. Season to taste.

2 Heat the butter in a small omelette or frying pan (skillet). Ideally this should be no larger than 12–15 cm (5–6 inches) in diameter. Too large a pan means the eggs are spread too thinly. Adding the oil is not essential but helps prevent the omelette sticking to the pan.

3 When the butter, or butter and oil, is hot pour in the eggs and cook over a moderate heat. Leave undisturbed for about 30 seconds to allow the omelette to begin to set on the underside.

4 This is the time to 'work' the omelette. Loosen the eggs from around the sides of the pan, then tilt it so that the still-liquid egg runs from the top to the sides of the pan. Do this until the omelette is set to your taste.

5 Fold or roll the omelette away from the handle, tip on to a hot plate and serve at once.

Variation

* To give a richer flavour and help prevent the omelette sticking to the pan, stir 1 (1¼) tablespoons of melted butter or olive oil into the eggs just before cooking.

Flavourings and Fillings

- Add a mixture of freshly chopped herbs to the eggs; this is known as *aux fine herbes.*

- *Cheese Omelette:* either add a small amount of grated cheese to the beaten eggs, or cover the top of the cooked omelette with grated cheese or spoonfuls of cheese before folding. For a main meal the omelette can be filled with a thick cheese sauce. Often this is mixed with lightly cooked vegetables.

- *Fish Omelette:* mix flaked, cooked fish with the beaten eggs and add chopped herbs to taste.

- *Mushroom Omelette:* either add finely diced, uncooked mushrooms to the beaten eggs, or fill the cooked omelette with small whole, or sliced, mushrooms of various kinds, precooked in a little oil or butter.

- *Prawn (Shrimp) Omelette:* either add a few spoonfuls of peeled and finely chopped cooked prawns (shelled shrimp) to the eggs, or heat whole prawns in a little hot butter and add to the omelette just before folding. If using frozen prawns defrost and dry well on paper towels before chopping or heating. (Avoid this omelette until you have finished the initial diet.)

- *Thai Omelette:* to give the eggs a taste of the Far East flavour them with a little finely chopped lemon grass and grated root ginger or ground ginger. Fill the cooked omelette with hot, crisp bean sprouts.

- *Tomato Omelette:* if you are satisfied that tomatoes do not adversely affect your arthritis fill the cooked omelette with thinly sliced, raw tomatoes or a thick tomato purée before folding.

- *Vegetable Omelette:* fill the cooked omelette with lightly cooked, diced root or other vegetables. (While on the diet avoid those in the nightshade family – listed page 57.)

Tortilla (Spanish Omelette)

This is a different kind of omelette, eaten cold as well as hot, and solid enough for a packed lunch. The traditional vegetables are potatoes and onions with perhaps a little chopped garlic. However, potatoes must be avoided during the initial days of the diet, so instead use rings of onion with sliced parsnips, carrots and sweet potato or yam, steamed or boiled in a very little salted water until just tender.

Strain well then heat in a little olive oil or oil and butter in the omelette or frying pan. Beat the eggs as instructed in step 1, pour over the hot vegetables and cook steadily until the eggs are set. Do not try and tilt the pan when making this omelette and do not fold. Simply slide onto a plate. Serve hot or cold cut into wedges.

Sweet Potato Rösti

Rösti is normally made with ordinary potatoes, but sweet potatoes or yams make an excellent alternative. The Swiss-inspired dish retains the full flavour of the vegetables, and is excellent served with main dishes. The chives or spring onions (scallions) are not essential, but give the sweet potatoes a more savoury flavour. Sweet potatoes and yams cook more rapidly than ordinary potatoes so do make sure they are not over-cooked before grating them. The steaming time will vary slightly according to the shape of the vegetables.

Sweet potatoes and yams can also be baked in their skins, boiled, mashed, fried and roasted just like ordinary potatoes. However, they have a fairly high sugar content so they burn more easily when roasted or fried.

Ingredients

SERVES 4

METRIC (IMPERIAL)	AMERICAN
450g (1lb) sweet potatoes or yams	1lb
3 tablespoons very finely chopped chives or spring onions (scallions)	3¾ tablespoons
sea salt and freshly ground black pepper to taste	

For frying
50g (2oz) butter	¼ cup
2 teaspoons sunflower or groundnut oil	2 teaspoons

Method

1 Scrub the potatoes or yams and place in a steamer. Cook for 6–8 minutes, or until the outsides begin to feel slightly softened.

2 Cool slightly, then remove the skins and rub the vegetables against a coarse grater. Let the flesh fall into a bowl as you do so. Mix in the chives or spring onions and a generous amount of seasoning.

3 Heat the butter and oil in a large frying pan (skillet). Add the potato mixture and spread out flat. Cook slowly for 7 minutes or until brown on the underside. Hold a large plate over the top of the frying pan and invert the pan so the rösti falls on to the plate with the browned side uppermost.

4 Slide the rösti back into the frying pan so the browned side is uppermost. Cook for 6–7 minutes, then tip on to a serving dish and cut into portions.

Variations

* Instead of one large potato cake make several smaller cakes, turning them over when browned on the under side, then cooking until brown on the second side.

* Use all sunflower or other oil instead of butter and a little oil.

* Parsnips and celeriac: both these vegetables make excellent rösti, either alone or mixed together.

* Peeled and grated raw vegetables can be used but this means a longer frying time and the need to use rather more butter and oil.

Freezing
Rösti freezes well.

Minted Beans and Cabbage

This satisfying blend of vegetables and apple could make a good vege-tarian main meal (see under Variations). It is also a good accompani-ment to liver.

In the initial stages of the diet it is recommended that as many vege-tables as possible are eaten raw. Undoubtedly there will be times when you would prefer hot vegetables; just make sure they are given the short-est possible cooking time, in the minimum of boiling water or, better still, that they are steamed. They will then retain the maximum vitamin and mineral content.

Often the thought of having several saucepans in use deters people from cooking a selection of vegetables, but if you cut them to a size that insures they need similar cooking times then they can be placed in one saucepan or steamer. Occasionally you will need to add vegetables at different times, as in the recipe below.

Ingredients

SERVES 4

METRIC (IMPERIAL)	AMERICAN
675–900g (1½–2lb) fresh broad (fava) beans*	1½–2lb
1 tablespoon olive oil	1¼ tablespoons
1 large onion, cut into rings	1
300ml (10fl oz) water	1¼ cups
sea salt and freshly ground black pepper to taste	
1 teaspoon grainy mustard	1 teaspoon
115g (4oz) courgettes (zucchini), cut into thin strips about 5cm (2 inches) long	¼lb
about ¼ red cabbage heart, finely shredded	about ¼
2 dessert apples, cored but not peeled, and thinly sliced	2
2 tablespoons chopped mint	2½ tablespoons

*You need about 350g (12oz/2¼ cups) after shelling.

Method

1 Remove the beans from the pods. Heat the oil in a saucepan, add the onion and sauté gently for 4 minutes. Pour in the water and add a little salt, pepper and the mustard. Bring to the boil.
2 Add the beans and cook steadily for 5 minutes, then put in the courgettes, cabbage and apples and continue cooking for 3–4 minutes. Stir in half the mint and strain. Keep the liquid as it makes a good vegetable stock (bouillon).
3 Spoon the mixture into a heated dish and top with the remaining mint.

Variations

❋ If the beans are very young they can be cooked in the pods; simply remove the ends. If you can do this allow only about 450g (1lb).
❋ Dried beans: when fresh broad beans are not in season make this dish with cooked dried beans. Remember that when cooking dried beans, especially red kidney beans, they must be given 10 minutes fast boiling during the cooking process, to remove toxins. Follow step 1, then add the beans with the courgettes and other ingredients.
❋ Canned beans: if using canned beans, rinse and drain them well. Add in step 2 after the vegetables and apples.
❋ For a main dish: add 225g (8oz/½ cup) diced tofu to the pan with the beans or top the cooked dish with mint and a thick layer of blanched, flaked almonds.

Do not freeze

Garlic Mushrooms

This dish can be served as a starter or light snack. There are many kinds of mushrooms on sale but I find that medium-sized button ones hold the garlic filling best.

Ingredients Serves 4–6 as a starter or 2–3 as a snack

Metric (Imperial)	American
450g (1lb) medium button or small cup mushrooms	1lb

For the filling

3–4 garlic cloves, peeled	3–4
115g (4oz) butter, slightly softened	½ cup
2 tablespoons very finely chopped parsley	2½ tablespoons
sea salt and freshly ground black pepper to taste	

Method

1 Finely chop or crush the garlic cloves. Mix with the butter, parsley and seasoning.
2 Remove the stalks from the mushrooms and keep them for making stock (bouillon). Wipe the caps well and place in an ovenproof dish with the stalk sides uppermost. Fill with the garlic mixture.
3 Preheat the oven to 200°C/400°F/Gas Mark 6 or 190°C for a fan (convection) oven. Bake for 10 minutes and serve hot with a green salad.

Variations

❋ Use other herbs, such as a mixture of chives, thyme and oregano instead of parsley.
❋ Cook in the microwave on High for about 6 minutes.
❋ *Cheese-topped Garlic Mushrooms:* when you can have a choice of cheese, cover the filled mushrooms with a thin layer of finely grated Cheddar or other good cooking cheese before baking.

Do not freeze

Avocado and Pineapple Salad

*This unusual salad not only makes a delicious start to a meal but can be
served equally well as a dessert (see under Variations).*

Ingredients

METRIC (IMPERIAL)	AMERICAN
For the dressing	
4 tablespoons single (light) cream	5 tablespoons
1 tablespoon cider or apple vinegar	1¼ tablespoons
1 tablespoon chopped coriander (cilantro)	1¼ tablespoons
For the salad	
4 slices fresh pineapple	4
2 ripe avocados	2
sea salt and freshly ground white pepper to taste	
rocket (arugula) leaves to taste	

Method

1   Mix together the ingredients for the dressing. It is important to have this ready before cutting the avocados, to prevent the fruit discolouring.
2   Remove the skin and centre hard core from the pineapple, then cut the rings into small neat portions. Add any juice that flows from the pineapple to the dressing.
3   Halve, peel and stone the avocados. Cut the flesh into neat dice or small balls with a vegetable scoop. Add to the dressing. Taste and add a very little seasoning if desired.
4   Arrange the rocket leaves on individual plates. Top with the avocado and dressing, then with the pineapple.

Variation

✤   To turn this into a dessert, use double (heavy) cream instead of single (light) cream. Sweeten this with a little clear honey and flavour it with a teaspoon of chopped mint. Omit the vinegar, coriander and seasoning. Stir the avocado into the cream. Spoon into individual glasses and top with diced pineapple and mint leaves.

Do not freeze

Buckwheat Salad

In spite of the name, buckwheat is not a wheat but a member of the rhubarb family. As it is filling it can take the place of potatoes while you are finding out if these have any adverse affect on your arthritis. It is an excellent ingredient in a salad. No cooking is required – just soften the grains with boiling liquid.

Ingredients

SERVES 4

METRIC (IMPERIAL)	AMERICAN
115g (4oz) coarse buckwheat	½ cup
300ml (10fl oz) water	1¼ cups
¼ teaspoon saffron strands or powder, optional	¼ teaspoon
2 pomegranates	2
mixed salad greens	
2 tablespoons Vinaigrette Dressing (see page 164)	2½ tablespoons
2 kiwi fruit	2

Method

1   Put the buckwheat into a bowl. Bring the water to the boil, add the saffron, if using, and pour over the buckwheat. Stir briskly, then leave until cold.
2   Strain the buckwheat, discarding the surplus moisture. Transfer to a large plate to dry out slightly.
3   Halve the pomegranates and scoop out the juicy seeds; mix with the buckwheat.
4   Arrange the salad greens on individual plates and sprinkle with the dressing. Make a neat mound of buckwheat in the middle. Peel and slice the kiwi fruits and arrange around the wheat.

Variations

❋ Instead of saffron use a little turmeric. This, like saffron, colours the grains and makes them look more attractive.
❋ If you find tomatoes have no adverse affect on your arthritis you could use freshly prepared tomato juice instead of water. Boil and use in the same way as the water. Omit the pomegranate seeds in this case and add finely diced cucumber instead.

Do not freeze

Fruit and Vegetable Salads

These simple salads can be served at any time of the day. They may well take the place of the biscuits you previously enjoyed midmorning or at tea time.

They make very good hors d'oeuvre at the start of a meal, or accompaniments to both hot and cold dishes.

Apple and Beetroot (Beet)

Mix equal quantities of peeled and diced cooked beetroot with peeled, cored and diced dessert apple. Add a few raisins and moisten with Vinaigrette Dressing (see page 164). Serve on watercress. This is particularly good with cold or hot duck. In this case, add finely chopped sage leaves.

Avocado, Celery and Cucumber

Pour 4 (5) tablespoons of Vinaigrette Dressing (see page 164) into a bowl. Halve, stone and peel 1 large or 2 small avocados. Cut the flesh into neat dice. Put into the dressing together with 6 (7½) tablespoons of finely diced celery heart and the same amount of unpeeled, thinly sliced cucumber. Serve on a bed of mixed lettuce leaves.

Green Bean, Apple and Pineapple

Cook diced green beans until tender. Strain and mix with equal amounts of unpeeled, diced dessert apple and diced fresh pineapple. Moisten with any pineapple juice that flows as you cut the fruit, and a very little extra virgin olive oil. Serve on a bed of rocket (arugula) and top with chopped walnuts. Red chillies make a colourful garnish if you find you can eat these.

Pear, Peach and Almond

Mix equal amounts of peeled, sliced dessert pears and peeled, halved and stoned ripe peaches. Make a dressing with a little apple vinegar, honey to sweeten and sea salt. Turn the fruits in this to moisten and retain their colour. Serve on a bed of shredded lettuce and top with whole blanched almonds.

Sweetcorn

Cook 2 large corn cobs, then strip away the kernels and put into 3 (3³/₄) tablespoons of Mayonnaise (see page 166) or yoghurt. Spoon on to a bed of lettuce and sliced cucumber and garnish with thin slices of ripe melon.

Do not freeze

Grilled Goat's Cheese Salad

*Combining hot ingredients with cold gives a modern touch to this salad.
It makes a good dinner-party dish as you can prepare the ingredients in
advance and assemble them while grilling (broiling) the cheese at the
last minute.*

Ingredients

METRIC (IMPERIAL)	AMERICAN
For the dressing	
3 tablespoons extra virgin olive oil	3¾ tablespoons
1½ tablespoons cider vinegar	2 tablespoons
1 teaspoon balsamic vinegar	1 teaspoon
2 teaspoons clear honey	2 teaspoons
1 garlic clove, finely chopped	1
2 teaspoons chopped oregano	2 teaspoons
1 teaspoon Dijon mustard	1 teaspoon
sea salt and freshly ground black pepper to taste	
For the salad	
2 celery sticks, chopped	2
2 dessert apples, peeled, cored and sliced	2
mixed salad greens, shredded	
For the cheese	
4 small individual goat's cheeses	4
1 tablespoon butter, melted	1¼ tablespoons

Method

1 Mix together the dressing ingredients. Add the celery and apple and leave to marinate for 30 minutes. Arrange the salad greens on individual plates and top with the celery, apple and dressing.
2 Place the cheeses under the preheated grill (broiler), brush with the butter and heat for 2–3 minutes or until the cheese is just starting to melt.
3 Spoon on to the salad and serve at once.

Do not freeze

Liver and Herb Salad

The liver for this salad can be grilled (broiled) or sautéed – see pages 132 and 134. Whichever method you choose, cut the still-warm cooked liver into narrow strips and marinate it in the dressing so it absorbs the flavour and becomes beautifully moist.

Ingredients

METRIC (IMPERIAL)	AMERICAN
2 slices of calves' or lambs' liver or about 4 chicken livers, cooked	2

For the dressing

2 tablespoons virgin olive oil	2½ tablespoons
1 tablespoon rice or red wine vinegar	1¼ tablespoons
½ teaspoon grated root ginger	½ teaspoon
1 teaspoon finely chopped lemon grass	1 teaspoon
2 teaspoons chopped basil	2 teaspoons
1 teaspoon chopped tarragon	1 teaspoon
1 teaspoon honey	1 teaspoon

For the salad

a few rocket (arugula) leaves	a few
a few watercress sprigs	a few
a few lettuce leaves	a few
1 or 2 fresh pineapple slices, diced	1 or 2

Method

1 Cut the cooked liver into narrow strips while still warm. Mix the ingredients for the dressing together and pour into a shallow casserole. Add the liver, cover and leave in the refrigerator for several hours or overnight.

2 Arrange the salad ingredients on a large plate. Scatter the strips of liver on top and sprinkle with the dressing.

Do not freeze

Mushroom and Liver Salad

The combination of hot mushrooms and a cold salad is very pleasant. Although the liver is given as cooked in the recipe you could have it uncooked if you enjoy it that way.

Ingredients

SERVES 1

METRIC (IMPERIAL)	AMERICAN
2 teaspoons olive oil	2 teaspoons
100g (3½oz) mushrooms, preferably chestnut, wiped and thickly sliced	1 cup
sea salt and freshly ground black pepper to taste	
100g (3½oz) cooked liver (see page 132), neatly diced	½ cup
2 tablespoons pine (pignolia) nuts	2½ tablespoons
green salad leaves to taste	
Vinaigrette Dressing (see page 164) to taste	

Method

1 Heat the oil in a frying pan (skillet) and cook the mushrooms for 5 minutes. Season to taste and keep warm while preparing the salad.

2 Mix the liver and nuts with the salad leaves and sprinkle with a little dressing. Pile on to a serving plate and top with the warm mushroom slices.

Variations

- Use cooked chicken livers and walnuts instead of mushrooms and pine nuts.
- Add a few tablespoons of alfalfa sprouts to the salad.
- Microwave: cook the mushrooms in just one teaspoon of oil in a bowl in the microwave for about 2 minutes.

Do not freeze

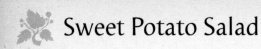

Sweet Potato Salad

Sweet potatoes or yams make a delicious and very satisfying salad. It is better to steam the vegetable before peeling as it will then be firmer and easier to dice neatly.

Ingredients

METRIC (IMPERIAL)	**AMERICAN**
For the dressing	
2 tablespoons olive oil	2½ tablespoons
2 tablespoons cider vinegar	2½ tablespoons
3 tablespoons single (light) cream	3¾ tablespoons
1 teaspoon clear honey	1 teaspoon
2 teaspoons chopped mint	2 teaspoons
2 teaspoons snipped chives	2 teaspoons
sea salt and freshly ground white pepper to taste	
For the salad	
1 large sweet potato	1
2 dessert apples, unpeeled but cored and sliced	2
salad greens to taste	

Method

1 Mix all the ingredients for the dressing together in a large bowl. Scrub the sweet potato, place in a steamer with a little salt and pepper and steam for about 8–10 minutes, or until tender but not over-soft.

2 Put the prepared apples into the dressing. Make sure it covers them completely, to prevent discolouration.

3 When the sweet potato is cooked, peel it and cut the flesh into neat small dice. Carefully stir into the dressing, taking care to keep the dice unbroken. Spoon the potato, apple and dressing mixture over the salad greens and serve.

Do not freeze

Main Dish Salads

It is important to have as many of the salad ingredients uncooked as possible. If you have not tried shredded raw spinach, Brussels sprouts and other green vegetables you will find their flavour unexpectedly delicious.

Try grated, raw root vegetables too – carrots are familiar but young celeriac, parsnips, turnips and swedes (rutabaga) are also excellent. A suitable dressing for these salads is found on page 164 and hints on varying this are given below. All these salads serve four.

Duck and Apple Salad

Remove the skin from a whole cooked bird or cooked duck portions, then cut the flesh into long narrow strips.

Make the Vinaigrette Dressing on page 164 and add to this a crushed garlic clove, 1–2 teaspoons of grated root ginger and 2 teaspoons of chopped sage leaves. Put the duck strips into the dressing and leave for 30 minutes.

Halve, but do not peel, 2 red-skinned dessert apples; remove the cores and cut each apple into about 8 slices. Add to the dressing together with 50g (2oz/$\frac{1}{3}$ cup) of raisins.

Prepare a large platter of shredded raw spinach, grated carrots, grated turnip and lightly cooked chopped green beans. Spoon the duck, apple and dressing on top.

Variations

Cooked chicken, pheasant or guinea fowl could be used instead of cooked duck. Substitute finely chopped rosemary for the sage.

Roquefort and Asparagus Salad*

If the asparagus is very young you could serve it raw, but most people prefer it lightly cooked. Put the asparagus into lightly salted water and cook for just a few minutes; the stalks should still be firm and a little crunchy. Drain carefully and arrange on a bed of sliced cucumber and shredded raw spinach.

*Do not serve this salad during the initial diet.

Make the Vinaigrette Dressing on page 164, then add 150g (5oz/1 cup) of finely diced Roquefort cheese and 2 (2½) tablespoons of snipped chives. Spoon over the salad.

Lentil and Pine (Pignolia) Nut Salad

Any kind of lentils can be used but the famous Puy type have the best flavour. First peel and chop 2 onions and 2 garlic cloves. Heat 2 (2½) tablespoons of olive oil in a large saucepan, add the onions and cook gently for 2 minutes, then put in the garlic and cook for a further 2 minutes.

Pour 600ml (1 pint/2½ cups) of water into the pan. Bring to the boil, then add 115g (4oz/½ cup) lentils together with a little sea salt and freshly ground black pepper. Cover the pan and cook steadily for 15–25 minutes until tender but still firm. Puy lentils take the longer time. Do not over-cook, the lentils should retain a firm texture.

If any liquid remains, drain well. Leave until cold, then stir in 2 peeled and finely chopped dessert apples or small ripe pears, 115g (4oz/1 cup) pine nuts, 2 (2½) tablespoons chopped parsley and 2 (2½) tablespoons finely snipped chives.

Mound the lentil mixture on individual plates and surround with a border of watercress and rocket (arugula) leaves. Spoon a little Vinaigrette Dressing over just before serving.

Variations

❋ *Bean and Walnut Salad:* use cooked borlotti (pinto) beans, or raw or lightly cooked broad (fava) beans when in season instead of lentils; and coarsely chopped walnuts instead of pine (pignolia) nuts.

❋ If you find you can eat tomatoes with no ill effect add 2 large peeled, deseeded and chopped tomatoes to the onions and garlic before adding the water.

Do not freeze

Apricot Rice Pudding

Rice is one of the familiar foods you can enjoy on your initial diet. Perhaps it is years since you made a rice pudding – now classed as old-fashioned. The recipe below brings the pudding up to date by using coconut milk and dried apricots, as well as the more conventional ingredients.

If you are allergic to cows' milk choose goats' or soya milk instead. I suggest sweetening the pudding with honey but other forms of sweetening are date syrup and agave syrup (both natural products), which are sold in health food stores. If you have none of these and use sugar, make sure it is natural (untreated) and organic.

Ingredients   SERVES 4

METRIC (IMPERIAL)	AMERICAN
115g (4oz) tenderized (ready to eat) dried apricots	¼lb
85g (3oz) raisins	½ cup
50g (2oz) short grain (pudding) rice	4 tablespoons
300ml (10fl oz) milk	1¼ cups
300ml (10fl oz) coconut milk	1¼ cups
1 tablespoon honey	1¼ tablespoons
150ml (5fl oz) apple juice	⅔ cup

Method

1   Preheat the oven to 150°C/300°F/Gas Mark 2 or 140°C for a fan (convection) oven.

2   Cut the apricots into small pieces. Put half of these and half the raisins into a 900–1200 ml (1½–2 pint/3¾–5 cup) pie or soufflé dish.

3   Rinse the rice in cold water and drain well. Add to the dried fruit together with the two kinds of milk and the honey. Stir gently to mix the ingredients and bake for 1½–2 hours. Reduce the heat slightly if the top of the pudding is becoming too brown. Stirring halfway through will help give a creamy texture.

4   Meanwhile, add the remaining apricots and raisins to the apple juice. Just before the pudding is ready, heat this mixture in a saucepan, or in a bowl in the microwave, until the fruit is well softened and most of the liquid has evaporated.

5   Serve topped with the hot apricot and raisin mixture.

Variation

✿ If more convenient bake the pudding in a slower oven, 140°C/275°F/Gas Mark 1 or 130°C for a fan (convection) oven.

Do not freeze

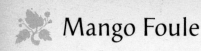

Mango Foule

I have used the original name for this dessert instead of the more familiar word 'fool'. It comes from the French verb fouler, meaning to chop, and the fruit should be finely diced rather than being made into a smooth purée. You can, of course, please yourself as to how you prepare it, but I think diced fruit makes the dessert seem more satisfying.

Ingredients

SERVES 4

METRIC (IMPERIAL)	AMERICAN
2 large ripe mangoes	2

For the custard

2 large eggs	2
300ml (10fl oz) milk	1¼ cups
2 teaspoons or to taste honey	2 teaspoons or to taste
150ml (5fl oz) double (heavy) cream or thick yoghurt	⅔ cup

To decorate

blanched almonds

Method

1   Cut a long slice from each side of the mango stones, scoop out the pulp from the slices and from around the stones. Chop finely.
2   Beat the eggs, add the milk and honey, then place the bowl over a pan of simmering water and whisk or stir briskly until the custard thickens.
3   Add the fruit to the warm custard and allow to cool.
4   Whip the cream until it just stands in peaks, then fold into the mango and custard mixture. Yoghurt will not need whipping.
5   Spoon into individual glasses and chill well. Top with the almonds and serve.

Variations

✻   Use other ripe fruit, such as peaches, nectarines and soft berries. Sieve the latter to remove the pips.
✻   Gooseberries make an excellent Fruit Foule; unless they are very ripe, cook them first in the minimum of water.

Freezing

It is better to sieve the fruit if you intend freezing the mixture.

Ginger and Lemon Pears

In this recipe the lemon flavour is provided by the use of lemon grass or the herb lemon balm. Keep the slices of root ginger fairly thick, so they are easy to remove. If you like a strong ginger taste grate the root finely so it becomes part of the sauce.

Ingredients

SERVES 4

METRIC (IMPERIAL)	AMERICAN
150ml (5fl oz) water	⅔ cup
3 tablespoons clear honey	3¾ tablespoons
2.5cm (1 inch) root ginger, peeled and sliced or grated (see above)	1 inch
1 lemon grass stalk or large sprig lemon balm	1
4 large dessert pears, halved, peeled and cored	4

Method

1 Pour the water into a large frying pan (skillet) or into a microwave-able bowl. Bring to the boil, then stir in the honey and ginger.

2 Strip and discard the outer skin from the lemon grass, then finely chop the stalk. If it seems tough then crush before chopping. Lemon balm should be washed and chopped. Add to the honey syrup.

3 *In a frying pan:* add the pear halves and simmer gently in the syrup for 10–15 minutes, depending on the ripeness of the fruit.

4 *In the microwave:* make the syrup in the bowl, then add the pear halves and give 5–8 minutes on High. Stand for 3 minutes before serving.

5 If you have used sliced ginger, remove it with a slotted spoon. Serve hot or cold.

Freezing
This dessert freezes well.

Peaches in Honey and Almonds

This is a delicious way of cooking peaches, whether they are just ripe or slightly under-ripe.

Ingredients

METRIC (IMPERIAL)	AMERICAN
4 large peaches, halved and stoned	4 large

For the sauce

6 tablespoons water	7½ tablespoons
2 tablespoons clear honey	2½ tablespoons

For the filling

50g (2oz) ground almonds	½ cup
1 tablespoon clear honey	1¼ tablespoons
25g (1oz) flaked blanched almonds	¼ cup

Method

1 Preheat the oven to 190°C/375°/Gas Mark 5 or 180°C for a fan (convection) oven.
2 Place the peaches in a large ovenproof dish with the cut sides uppermost.
3 Heat the water with the honey in a saucepan or in a bowl in the microwave. Pour over and around the peaches.
4 Mix the ground almonds and honey together and place a little in each peach half. Stud with the almonds.
5 Cover the dish with a lid or foil and bake for 15–25 minutes, depending on the ripeness of the peaches. For a slightly browned effect, remove the foil for the last 3 minutes of cooking. Serve hot or cold.

Variation

✳ When fresh peaches are not in season use canned peaches in natural juice, well drained. The juice can be used instead of water to make the filling.

Do not freeze

Summer Soufflé Omelette

A light fluffy omelette filled with seasonal fruit (as shown on the cover) makes an attractive and nourishing dessert. The filling can be varied throughout the year.

You are advised to avoid sugar as much as possible, particularly during the early stages of the diet, and use honey. Unfortunately this makes the eggs too sticky and spoils the lightness of the omelette, so use sugar for this purpose. If possible, choose sugar that is both natural and organic.

Ingredients   SERVES 2

METRIC (IMPERIAL)	AMERICAN
For the fruit filling	
150ml (5fl oz) water	⅔ cup
1 tablespoon honey or sugar	1¼ tablespoons
225g (8oz) mixed summer fruits (raspberries, red and black currants, cherries)	½lb
For the omelette	
4 large eggs	4
2 tablespoons caster (superfine) sugar	2½ tablespoons
a few drops vanilla extract	a few drops
1 tablespoon single (light) cream or milk	1¼ tablespoons
25g (1oz) butter	2 tablespoons
To decorate	
a little icing (confectioner's) sugar	a little
large sprig of mint	

Method

1 Put the water into a saucepan with the honey or sugar. Bring to the boil and simmer for 3 minutes, then remove from the heat. Add the fruits and allow to stand. This prevents the soft fruits being over-cooked but allows the syrup to flavour and slightly soften them.

2 Separate the eggs and lightly beat the yolks with the sugar, vanilla and cream or milk. Whisk the egg whites in a separate bowl until they stand in soft peaks, then fold into the yolks.

3 Preheat the grill (broiler) on a medium setting. Heat the butter in an omelette or frying pan (skillet), pour in the egg mixture and cook steadily until the bottom of the omelette is set; the top should still be runny.

4 Place the pan under the grill and cook until the egg mixture is just set. Cover half the omelette with the warm fruit, fold the other half over it and slide on to a heated dish.

5 Sift over a little icing sugar, top with the mint and serve at once.

Do not freeze

Strawberry and Grape Sorbet

Sorbets (sherbets) can be made with almost any fruit. If the fruit itself is not very juicy you can add liquid in the form of apple, grape or pineapple juice. If you find you are not allergic to citrus fruits then lemon, lime or orange juices give wonderful flavours to sorbets.

One of the primary objects of this book is to ensure that people with arthritis are eating helpful foods. So many commercially made products include such a wide range of added ingredients that it is difficult to ascertain just what may, or may not, be affecting your arthritis. If you make your own sorbets and ice cream (see page 210) then you know exactly what is in them.

Ingredients   SERVES 4–6

METRIC (IMPERIAL)	AMERICAN
450g (1lb) strawberries	1lb
250ml (8fl oz) grape juice	1 cup
1 tablespoon or to taste honey	1¼ tablespoons or to taste

Method

1 Put all the ingredients into a liquidizer or food processor and process until smooth. The small seeds in strawberries are generally crushed after this, but if you want an absolutely smooth liquid then pass it through a sieve.

2 *With an ice-cream maker:* pour the mixture into the container, switch on until sufficiently aerated and frosted, then spoon into a suitable container and store in the freezer.

3 *Without an ice-cream maker:* pour the mixture into freezing trays and place in the freezer until lightly frosted. Turn into a bowl, whisk briskly to aerate the mixture, then return to the trays or a suitable container and continue freezing. This stage of whisking is not essential but it gives a better texture; see also under Variations.

4 Always bring a sorbet out of the freezer about 15 minutes before serving. Store in the refrigerator, then spoon into chilled glasses or dishes.

Variations

❦ Use any fruits or combinations of fruits. If you have a juice extractor you can also freeze vegetable juices (without sweetening) or combine them with fruit juices.

❦ It is possible to lighten the fruit mixture by incorporating egg whites at step 2. This is not necessary if you have an ice cream maker but a good idea (if you do not mind eating uncooked egg whites) when making sorbets by hand. Whisk the whites of 2 large eggs until stiff, then fold into the half-frozen mixture at step 2.

Vanilla Ice Cream

Ice cream should be omitted during the initial stages of the diet and even after that it is better to make your own, unless you can buy organic ice cream that does not contain additives that could affect your arthritis. The first recipe is based on a classic method of making the dessert but it is high in both fat and calories. It does, however, produce a wonderfully smooth result, even if frozen in an ordinary freezer or freezing compartment of the refrigerator. If you want to produce low-fat and low-calorie ice cream regularly you would be well-advised to purchase an ice cream maker. Some are now quite inexpensive.

If you are allergic to cows' milk, try using goats' milk, ewes' milk or soya milk, or use tofu (bean curd) as suggested opposite.

Ingredients

SERVES 4–6

METRIC (IMPERIAL)	AMERICAN
300ml (10fl oz) milk	1¼ cups
2 yolks from large eggs (or 2 whole eggs)	2
1 tablespoon or to taste honey or organic caster (superfine) sugar	1 tablespoon or to taste
1 vanilla pod (bean)	1
300ml (10fl oz) double (heavy) cream	1¼ cups

Method

1 Warm the milk but do not allow it to boil. Whisk the egg yolks or whole eggs with the honey or sugar, then add the milk.
2 Slit the vanilla pod, remove the seeds and add them to the egg mixture. (Save the pod and place it in a jar of sugar to flavour it.)
3 Pour the custard into a bowl or the top of a double saucepan and whisk or stir over hot, but not boiling, water until the mixture coats the back of a wooden spoon.

4   Place a piece of damp greaseproof paper or baking parchment over the custard to prevent a skin forming and leave until cold.

5   Whip the cream until it stands in soft peaks (do not over-whip), then fold into the custard. Spoon into a suitable container, cover and freeze. For a lighter texture freeze lightly then whisk to aerate and continue freezing.

Variations

* Use ½–1 teaspoon of vanilla extract instead of the vanilla seeds.
* *Low-fat Vanilla Ice Cream:* use single (light) cream or fromage frais instead of the double cream. Eat the ice cream when it has been freshly frozen, otherwise icicles form in the low-fat mixture. This is excellent if frozen in an ice cream maker.
* In an ice cream maker you can follow the basic recipe but use single (light) cream instead of the whipped double (heavy) cream.
* *Tofu Ice Cream:* if you are allergic to dairy products use tofu (bean curd). Buy the silken (soft) variety and either whisk or liquidize it to give a smoother texture. To 400g (14oz/good ¾lb) of tofu use the vanilla seeds, as suggested in step 2 opposite, or ½–1 teaspoon vanilla extract with honey or sugar to sweeten. Freeze lightly, then whisk to aerate and complete freezing. I find Tofu Ice Cream is better with a fruit flavour. Use about 200ml (7fl oz/scant 1 cup) of fruit purée to the 400g (14oz/2 cups) of tofu.
* *Fruit Ice Cream:* use the basic recipe with about 300ml (½ pint/1¼ cups) of your favourite fruit purée. Add to the custard and cream mixture.
* *Spiced Ice Cream:* flavour the ice cream with a little ground ginger or cinnamon.

Freezing

Store in the freezer but remove about 10 minutes before serving.

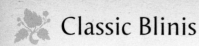

Classic Blinis

This recipe uses fine buckwheat flour. If you can obtain only coarse buckwheat and are using the American measures, use just 1 US cup and put into a food processor for a short time to make it finer.

Ingredients

METRIC (IMPERIAL)	AMERICAN
225g (8oz) fine buckwheat flour	2 cups
¼ teaspoon sea salt	¼ teaspoon
1 teaspoon easy-bake (instant) yeast	1 teaspoon
375ml (12½fl oz) milk	1½ cups
1 teaspoon clear honey	1 teaspoon
3 tablespoons double (heavy) cream	3¾ tablespoons
1 tablespoon butter, melted	1¼ tablespoons
2 large eggs	2

For cooking

a little sunflower oil, see step 8	a little
1 tablespoon butter, melted	1¼ tablespoons

Method

1 Mix the buckwheat flour, salt and easy-bake yeast together in a mixing bowl.

2 Warm the milk to blood heat (just comfortably warm), add to the flour and mix well.

3 Blend the honey with the cream and melted butter. Separate the eggs, add the yolks to the honey mixture, then stir into the mixing bowl.

4 Beat well for 3 minutes, then cover the bowl and put in a warm place for about 45 minutes or until almost doubled in bulk.

5 Beat the batter until smooth. Whisk the egg whites until stiff, then fold into the batter.

6 Heat 1 teaspoon of oil in a small pancake pan (skillet). Spoon in a little of the mixture to give a thickish pancake. Cook steadily for 2–3 minutes or until golden brown on the underside.

7 Turn over and brush the top of the pancake with a little of the melted butter. Cook for the same time on the second side.

8 Continue in this way. If using a non-stick pan you may not need any more extra oil but make sure the pan is well heated before cooking each pancake.

9 Serve hot with savoury or sweet ingredients.

Freezing
Separate each cooked pancake with squares of waxed paper. Defrost at room temperature.

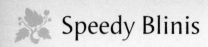 Speedy Blinis

The recipe for Classic Blinis, made with yeast, is on page 212. The recipe below uses the buckwheat in a quicker method. You will find these pancakes invaluable while you are avoiding ordinary wheat. They are delicious hot or cold. This recipe assumes you are using the coarser buckwheat. If you can obtain the finer buckwheat flour use 1 American cup and not ¾ cup, and don't liquidize the ingredients.

Ingredients

MAKES 8–10

METRIC (IMPERIAL)	**AMERICAN**
115g (4oz) coarse buckwheat flour	¾ cup
½ teaspoon sea salt	½ teaspoon
225ml (7½fl oz) water	scant 1 cup
2 large eggs, whisked	2
1 tablespoon, or as required oil*, optional	1¼ tablespoons, or as required

For cooking	
1 tablespoon oil*	1¼ tablespoons

*I like olive oil in the pancakes and groundnut or sunflower oil for cooking them

Method

1   Put the buckwheat and salt into a bowl. Bring the water to the boil, pour over the buckwheat and leave until cold.

2   Stir in the eggs and mix thoroughly. Add the oil just before cooking the pancakes. (This is not essential but helps stop the pancakes sticking and is invaluable if they are to be frozen.)

3   To give a smoother texture pour the ingredients into a liquidizer or food processor and process for about ½ minute. You will still have the nutty grains of the wheat but they will be finer.

4   Pour about 1 teaspoon of oil into a pancake pan (skillet) then add a large spoonful of the mixture. The ideal size for general purposes is about 10cm (4 inches) across. If necessary, spread out the mixture to give this size using the back of the spoon.

5   Cook over a low heat for 4–5 minutes, or until the pancake is golden brown on the underside and can be turned over easily. If you have a large pan, cook more than one at a time.

6   Continue in this way. If using a non-stick pan you may not need any more oil but make sure it is very hot before cooking each pancake.

7   Serve hot with savoury or sweet ingredients.

Freezing

Separate each cooked pancake with squares of waxed paper. Defrost at room temperature.

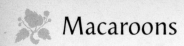

Macaroons

As macaroons contain a high percentage of sugar they should not be eaten regularly, but I feel that a treat now and again helps one to maintain a fairly strict regime. I have tested the macaroons with the amount of sugar given below, which is slightly less than usual, and they still have a very good flavour. To insure a sticky texture in the middle put a small ovenproof bowl or tin of water into the oven under the baking sheets.

Ingredients

MAKES 15

METRIC (IMPERIAL)	AMERICAN
a few sheets rice paper	a few sheets
2 whites from large eggs	2
a few drops almond extract	a few drops
150g (5oz) ground almonds	1¼ cups
115g (4oz) caster (superfine) sugar	½ cup

To decorate

15 blanched almonds	15

Method

1   Place the rice paper on 2 or 3 large baking sheets. Preheat the oven to 180°C/350°F/Gas Mark 4 or 170°C for a fan (convection) oven.

2   Whisk the egg whites until just frothy, then stir in the remainder of the ingredients. Divide into 15 small portions and roll these into balls. If the mixture seems a little sticky chill for a time in the refrigerator or dampen your fingertips before rolling them. Alternatively, just use spoonfuls of the mixture.

3   Place on the rice paper, allowing at least 3.75cm (1½ inches) around each macaroon as the mixture spreads during cooking. Press an almond into the middle of each macaroon.

4   Bake for 20 minutes or until evenly golden. Cool slightly, then remove from the baking sheets and cut around the rice paper.

5   The macaroons can be stored for a day in an airtight tin but they lose their texture and tend to crumble if kept longer.

Variation

* *Coconut Macaroons:* use 65g (2½oz/good ½ cup) ground almonds and 65g (2½oz/½ cup) desiccated (shredded) coconut.

Freezing

Macaroons can be frozen for about 2 weeks; after that they tend to crumble badly when removed from the freezer.

Millet Porridge

You may be able to buy gluten-free breakfast cereals from health food shops but it is easy to prepare a hot or cold breakfast dish with millet. This is a very nutritious grain. Porridge made with millet is familiar in many parts of the world.

The quantities below give one large or two small helpings.

Ingredients

SERVES 1 OR 2

METRIC (IMPERIAL)	AMERICAN
For preparation	
115g (4oz) millet	½ cup
4 tablespoons milk or water	5 tablespoons
For breakfast	
4 tablespoons or amount preferred milk	5 tablespoons or amount preferred
¼ teaspoon ground cinnamon (optional)	¼ teaspoon
amount required honey	amount required

Method

1 Put the millet into a bowl. Bring the milk or water to boiling point and pour over the millet. If you like crisp grains allow to stand for 10 minutes; to give a softer texture cover the bowl and leave in the refrigerator overnight.

2 Tip the mixture into a saucepan or microwaveable bowl and stir in the extra milk and the cinnamon, if using.

3 Heat well, then spoon into one or two serving dishes and top with honey.

Variations

✿ Add 3 (3¾) tablespoons of raisins at step 3.

✿ *Millet Muesli:* follow step 1. At breakfast time mix 2 (2½) tablespoons raisins, 1 or 2 unpeeled grated apples and 2 (2½) tablespoons of chopped walnuts with the millet. Spoon into one or two serving dishes and top with honey and yoghurt.

Do not freeze

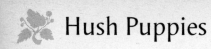

Hush Puppies

These fried corn cakes are an American speciality. They are ideal as a quick breakfast dish or as an accompaniment to savoury dishes.

All grains vary in the amount of liquid they absorb, so it is important to check the consistency at step 3.

When frying, be selective about the oil you use; discard stale oil that has been used on a number of occasions. A wok is good as you need less oil than in a frying pan (skillet) or deep fryer.

Ingredients

MAKES ABOUT 12

METRIC (IMPERIAL)	**AMERICAN**
115g (4oz) yellow or white maize (corn) meal	1 cup
1 teaspoon baking powder	1 teaspoon
½–1 teaspoon sea salt	½–1 teaspoon
1 teaspoon honey	1 teaspoon
1 tablespoon olive oil	1¼ tablespoons
2 large eggs	2
4 tablespoons or as required milk	5 tablespoons or as required
2 teaspoons chopped or grated onion or snipped chives	2 teaspoons

For frying

at least 250ml (8fl oz) vegetable oil	at least 1 cup

Method

1 Sift the maize meal, baking powder and salt into a mixing bowl.
2 Beat the honey, olive oil and eggs together. Add to the maize meal.
3 Gradually beat the milk into the other ingredients. The mixture should be the consistency of a thick batter that drops easily from a tablespoon but holds its shape. Stir in the onion or chives.
4 Pour the oil into a wok or frying pan (skillet). You need a depth of about 5cm (2 inches). Heat to a temperature of 170°C (340°F). To test without a thermometer drop in a cube of day-old bread; it should turn golden in 1 minute.
5 Drop in tablespoons of the mixture and fry for about 1½ minutes, or until golden. Turn over and cook for 1½ minutes on the second side, then lower the heat and cook more slowly for 2 minutes.
6 Lift the Hush Puppies out of the oil, drain on kitchen towels and serve hot.

Do not freeze

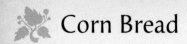

Corn Bread

Classic recipes for corn bread loaves are made with two parts maize (corn) meal to one part wheat flour. As that is not possible while avoiding wheat, the following soft bread is the best to bake. This is better eaten hot when freshly baked but it can be cooled, then cut into squares and reheated for a few minutes in the oven. Alternatively, toast it under a preheated grill (broiler) and use as a base for poached or scrambled eggs.

Ingredients

MAKES ABOUT 9 SQUARES

METRIC (IMPERIAL)	AMERICAN
115g (4oz) yellow or white maize (corn) meal	1 cup
1 teaspoon baking powder	1 teaspoon
½–1 teaspoon or to taste sea salt	½–1 teaspoon to to taste
40g (1½oz) butter, melted	3 tablespoons
2 teaspoons honey	2 teaspoons
125ml (4fl oz) water, boiling	½ cup
125ml (4fl oz) milk	½ cup
3 large eggs	3

Method

1 Preheat the oven to 190°C/375°F/Gas Mark 5 or 180°C for a fan (convection) oven. Line a 20cm (8 inch) square cake pan with baking parchment or grease thoroughly. (As the mixture is very liquid do not choose a pan with a loose base.)

2 Sift the maize meal, baking powder and salt into a mixing bowl. Mix the butter and honey with the boiling water, then add the cold milk.

3 Separate the eggs and whisk the yolks into the water and milk. Gradually beat into the maize meal.

4 Whisk the egg whites until they stand in soft peaks, then fold into the batter.

5 Pour into the prepared cake pan and bake for 35–40 minutes until golden brown and firm to a gentle pressure.

6 Cool in the pan for 5 minutes, then turn out on to a wire cooling tray.

Freezing

Replace in the cake pan. When cold, cut into squares and freeze. This means you can remove any number of squares as required. When frozen place in a container and cover.

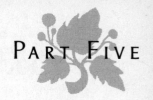

PART FIVE

Taking It Further

CHAPTER 1

Foods that heal

Many foods have healing qualities that can help arthritis sufferers. Try including the following ingredients in your cooking whenever possible.

Almonds – a rich source of calcium.

Angelica – a tall robust plant that has spread across Europe as a weed. Candied stalks are used in decorating cakes and other sweets. Toss young leaf shoots with salad greens and serve with a dressing of olive oil and concentrated apple juice.

Avocados – a good source of the omega-6 essential fatty acid, linoleic acid. Some nutritionists believe these delicious fruits also contain a substance that helps the elimination of uric acid from the body.

Bananas – a rich source of potassium, a mineral needed for the balance of fluids in the body, the transmission of nerve impulses, and muscle function. As you drink water, potassium is flushed from your body. Bananas are filling, come in a safe natural wrapper, are easy to digest and rarely cause food sensitivity.

Black pepper – improves circulation and thus helps control inflammation.

Black treacle (molasses) – rich in iron, potassium, magnesium and calcium, this sweet food should be taken daily and is an important part of the *Eat to Beat Arthritis* Diet.

Brazil nuts – an excellent source of selenium, and also S-adenosyl-methionine [SAMe], a chemical with pain-relieving properties similar to ibuprofen. Sunflower seeds also contain SAMe. As the quantities of SAMe are small, eat these foods as frequently as possible (you would need to eat about 250g (9oz) of Brazil nuts, or 500g (18oz) of sunflower seeds to receive the same benefit as from a single dose of a SAMe dietary supplement.) James A. Duke, Ph.D., author of *The Green Pharmacy*, said 'It is not feasible to eat that many nuts and seeds, but I believe that every little bit helps ...'

Brewers' yeast – taken daily as part of the *Eat to Beat Arthritis* Diet, this is an excellent source of folate and other members of the B-vitamin family, as well as the minerals iron, copper, phosphate, magnesium and zinc. It is an excellent natural supplement to promote healthy bones, joints and muscles.

Broccoli – a good source of glutathione, a powerful natural antioxidant that is thought to be beneficial in controlling symptoms of arthritis.

Camomile – used since the time of the ancient Egyptians to aid healing. Tea made with camomile calms the nerves and reduces stress. As stress promotes pain, sipping a warm cup of camomile tea in the evening helps you relax before going to bed.

Carrots – a rich source of beta-carotene, a precursor molecule the body turns into vitamin A. Beta-carotene is a powerful antioxidant. It is best consumed as a natural part of food, rather than as a manufactured dietary supplement. Other good food sources include sweet potatoes, apricots, mangoes and watercress.

Celery – contains compounds that help the body eliminate uric acid. Also contains an anti-inflammatory substance. Include raw celery in your diet at least three times a week, and use crushed celery seeds to top salads and savoury baked products.

Cherries – although there is no real scientific proof, some scientists claim that a substance in cherries helps the body eliminate uric acid.

Chilli peppers – capsaicin, a substance found in hot peppers, triggers the release of the body's own opiates, known as endorphins. Red peppers also contain salicylates, compounds that are closely related to aspirin. After you have tested your sensitivity to members of the nightshade family, try adding some peppers to your diet for healing as well as for flavour.

Fish – enjoy fresh fish rich in omega-3 fatty acids, such as mackerel, tuna, salmon and albacore. Fish eat green water plants that contain small amounts of linoleic acid. The body of the fish transforms this vital nutrient into DHA and EPA, which are then stored in the body fat of the animal. Some experts believe that eating foods rich in omega-3 fatty acids reduces the need for certain prescription medicines. Talk to your doctor about this after you have established your new diet programme.

Ginger – helps relieve the pain associated with inflammation, and stimulates the circulatory system. Combine with coriander in curries and sauces for meat. Jean Carper, author of *Food: Your Miracle Medicine*, drinks ginger tea for her osteoarthritis.

Liver – a rich source of B-vitamins and many of the minerals necessary for muscle, bone and joint health. (People with gout should avoid liver, however.) It is an excellent source of iron. Calves' liver has the best flavour.

Offal – this term refers to a number of internal organs eaten as meat, including liver, kidney, tripe and sweetbreads. High in protein, offal also contains significant amounts of key nutrients including the B-vitamins and minerals. As the liver is the most biologically (metabolically) active organ in the body, it is also the richest in those nutrients needed for normal human health and development. In terms of nutrient value, kidney and sweetbreads rank second and third. Tripe is a muscle, and has little value other than as a source of protein.

Olives – have had a reputation as a mild diuretic, a useful characteristic in the control of gout. There is some evidence from Japan that the daily consumption of about a quart (litre) of tea made from olive leaves increases the daily output of urine by 10–15 per cent, thus helping the body rid itself of uric acid.

Oregano – contains rosmarinic acid, which research has shown has powerful properties as an antioxidant, anti-viral, antibacterial and anti-inflammatory substance. Infused in combination with members of the mint family, oregano makes a satisfying and useful tea for arthritis sufferers. The pizza and pasta herbs – basil, marjoram and rosemary – all contain antioxidants that research suggests have anti-arthritic properties, so top up your food with flavours from the Mediterranean.

Parsley – used for centuries as a natural diuretic, it aids the elimination of uric acid from the body. Parsley is also a rich source of iron and vitamin C.

Pineapple – research suggests that bromelain, a substance found in fresh pineapple but not in canned, helps prevent inflammation and improve healing. This fruit also contains substances that block the formation of cancer-causing nitrosamines in the stomach.

Tea (green) – is the only caffeinated drink of potential benefit for people with bone disease. All tea contains isoflavonoids, which have a weak oestrogenic activity thought to protect bones against mineral loss, but their concentration in green tea is greater than in black tea. Recent scientific studies compared the bone-mineral density of women between the ages of 65 and 76 years who were either tea drinkers or non-tea drinkers. Statistically excluding factors such as HRT, smoking and coffee-drinking, the bone mineral density of tea drinkers was approximately 5% greater than that in women who drank no tea.

Turmeric – contains a useful substance that aids the pain of chronic arthritis. Curcumin, which gives the spice its brilliant yellow colour, is thought to block a neurotransmitter involved in carrying pain signals to various parts of the body. Curcumin also acts as an antioxidant, an antimicrobial and an anti-inflammatory.

According to Susan Clark, British Health Journalist of the Year and *Sunday Times* expert on alternative medicine, curcumin may work as well as the steroid cortisone in relieving acute inflammation. The recommended dose is 400–600mg per day. Turmeric contains between 0.3 and 5.4 per cent curcumin, so either prepare to eat large amounts of yellow food, or use a food supplement containing this substance. No toxic level has been established for curcumin, but it is always unwise to exceed recommended amounts of any supplement.

Walnuts – are good plant sources of omega-3 fatty acids. There is evidence that eating an ounce of walnuts three or four times a week can help reduce blood cholesterol levels.

Some important food tips

* Other foods supply specific nutrients that help combat arthritis. For example, avocados, peaches, watermelons, cabbage and cauliflower are all good sources of glutathione, a natural antioxidant which has been linked with arthritis. People who have low levels of this substance in their bodies are more likely to have arthritis. Asparagus and citrus fruit are also are good sources of glutathione, but do not include these in your diet until after you have tested your sensitivity to them (see pages 73–75). Asparagus is high in purines, substances which can increase the level of uric acid in the blood, and so should be avoided by those with gout. If you suffer from arthritis, try this vegetable after Week Two.

* Remember: if you are taking aspirin on a regular basis to cope with the pain of arthritis, eat plenty of vitamin C-rich foods. Aspirin destroys significant quantities of vitamin C.

* If you love the cheerful pink colour and sweet-sour taste of rhubarb, remember that it contains oxalate, a substance that interferes with the absorption of calcium needed for strong bones. Enjoy rhubarb in limited quantities.

Questions and answers about arthritis

What is arthritis?

Arthritis is a general term used to describe any disease or illness that causes inflammation of one or more joints. More than one hundred conditions are classified as arthritis by the medical profession. Some have names we recognize at once: rheumatoid arthritis, osteoarthritis and gout are examples. However, most forms of arthritis are relatively rare and receive limited public notice; these include carpal tunnel syndrome, ankylosing spondylosis, scleroderma, Lyme disease and systemic lupus.

What is a joint?

Joints are structures that occur where two bones meet. There are several types of joints: some allow movement while others do not. For example,

Articular joint

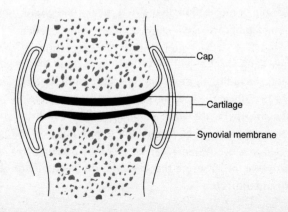

Cap

Cartilage

Synovial membrane

joints linking bones in the arms and legs move, but those between the flat bones of the skull do not. Most joints contain a cartilage pad at the end of each bone, a fibrous capsule, a lining of synovial membrane, a space partially filled with fluid secreted by the membrane, and ligaments. Fibrous connective tissue links bones in immobile joints.

Mobile joints, also known as synovial joints, are found in the jaw, spine, arms, shoulders, hands, hips, legs and feet. They are characterized by a fibrous wall lined with a thin sac that secretes a lubricating substance known as synovial fluid. These joints also contain cartilage pads at the end of adjoining bones; these act as shock absorbers during physical activity.

What is osteoarthritis?

The rubbery tissue (cartilage) covering the ends of bones meeting inside synovial joints is damaged by osteoarthritis (OA), leading to pain during movement. Abnormal spurs of bone may grow inside the damaged joint and add to discomfort. Although the exact cause of OA is unclear, the following are important risk factors:

* Joint injuries – caused by sports injuries or physical labour.
* Gender – women are affected more often than men.
* Age – people over 45 are at greatest risk.
* Inherited conditions affecting the joints or cartilage.
* Excess body weight.
* Any disease, or medication, that affects the normal production and function of joint cartilage.

It is most likely that OA will affect the fingers, spine and weight-bearing joints, including those in the hips, knees and feet. Swelling may occur, especially in the knee joints.

Osteoarthritis is the most common form of arthritis. It rarely develops before the age of 40 and almost everyone over the age of 75 is affected to some degree. It can be very mild, causing only an occasional twinge, or so severe that even the simplest activities become painful and difficult.

What is rheumatoid arthritis?

Rheumatoid arthritis (RA) is a chronic inflammatory disease that most commonly affects the synovial lining of joints; it can also cause inflammation of the lining surrounding the lungs and heart, and the membranes lining blood vessels. RA is caused by the body's own immune system attacking normal tissue. If the attack continues untreated over a long period of time, the cartilage and bony parts of joints may be destroyed. Individual cases vary widely in severity, however.

About one per cent of the world's population suffer from RA: every ethnic group is affected. Two to three times more women than men develop RA, and some experts believe hormones may be a factor because the risk decreases after the menopause. Genetics also plays a role in susceptibility to this condition and close relatives of people affected by RA are at risk of developing it. Siblings of RA patients have the highest risk of developing the disease.

Unlike other forms of arthritis, RA is symmetrical, attacking the same joints on both sides of the body. An attack can be extremely painful. Membranes surrounding a joint becomes inflamed, thickened, and produce an excessive amount of fluid. The build-up of this fluid produces pressure on the soft tissues surrounding the joint and damages the soft cartilage 'cushions' within the joint. The disease progresses at different rates, and its severity usually waxes and wanes over a number of years. RA will go into remission in a few people, usually within the first two years.

RA most commonly attacks the joints of the hands and feet, causing tenderness, swelling and pain. Generalized stiffness on getting out of bed in the morning is common. Usually late in the course of the disease, one in four RA patients develop hard *rheumatoid nodules* under their skin on the elbows, heels, hips, back of the head, fingers and toes.

What is gout?

Gout is a form of arthritis that occurs when crystals of uric acid accumulate in soft tissues, such as the kidneys and the joints of the feet and hands. The big toe is most frequently affected. Uric acid is a natural by-product of metabolism that is normally excreted in the urine. Gout occurs when the kidneys do not function adequately to remove uric acid from the body, or when the diet contains excessive quantities of foods containing substance called *purines* (proteins primarily found in the nucleus of cells). In both cases, the level of uric acid in the blood reaches abnormal concentrations and crystals of sodium biurate begin to form in soft tissues and joints. The crystal deposits grow for as long as the condition remains untreated.

Diet plays an important role in controlling this form of arthritis, and certain foods, including red meat, shellfish, anchovies, sardines, liver and sweetbreads should be avoided. The risk of an attack is increased by the excessive consumption of alcohol.

Gout tends to run in families, and men are more susceptible than women. Diabetes, high blood pressure and obesity are important risk factors.

What medications and treatments are used for the various forms of arthritis?

Osteoarthritis

The two most commonly prescribed treatments for OA are corticosteroids and non-steroidal anti-inflammatory drugs (NSAIDs), such as aspirin, ibuprofen and fenbufen. These work by blocking the action of specific hormone-like substances (prostaglandins), which are responsible for producing inflammation and, therefore, pain. Medications such as Tylenol and paracetamol relieve pain but do not reduce inflammation.

Recent scientific research demonstrates that glucosamine, a naturally occurring substance in the body, can reverse the damaging processes that destroy cartilage in the joints (see page 237).

Rheumatoid arthritis

Anti-rheumatic drugs are designed to relieve pain and stiffness, maintain mobility and prevent deformation of joints affected by rheumatic disorders. Three types of anti-rheumatic drugs are available:

- those that relieve symptoms;
- those that slow or halt the underlying condition causing the symptoms;
- corticosteroids.

Drugs used to reduce symptoms are usually prescribed as a first line of treatment, and include aspirin and non-steroidal anti-inflammatory drugs (NSAIDs) such as acemetacin, benorylate, diflunisal, fenbufen, fenoprofen, ibuprofen, mefenamic acid and tolmetin. They are called 'non-steroidal' to separate them from corticosteroid drugs, which also reduce inflammation. Although NSAIDs do nothing to stop the progress of the illness, they effectively reduce pain, swelling and stiffness that result from tissue inflammation. However, because the damage to joints remains, symptoms may recur.

If symptoms increase, drugs are prescribed which slow further damage to joints and tissues. These include:

- gold-based drugs, such as auranofin;
- immunosuppressants, such as azathioprine and chlorambucil;
- chloroqine and hydroxychloroquine;
- penicillamine (which is not an antibiotic);
- sulphasalazine.

Corticosteroids control pain by blocking the biochemical processes that trigger inflammation. These drugs are used for short periods of time because they temporarily depress the immune system. All anti-rheumatic drugs should be used under medical supervision to control side effects, some of which can be distressing.

Gout
Drugs used to prevent gout lower blood levels of uric acid. These include allopurinol, probenecid and sulphinpyrazone. Those prescribed to treat gout include NSAIDs and colchicine.

Which dietary supplements are helpful in treating arthritis?

FISH OIL

For decades, arthritis sufferers have experienced less pain and debilitating illness when they supplemented their diet with fish oil. No one knew why this was, and some medical experts doubted that the improvement was real and not simply a placebo effect. At the turn of this century, scientists at Cardiff University conducted a series of experiments exposing the cells responsible for the growth and repair of joint cartilage, called chondrocytes, to various mixtures of fatty acids. Not surprisingly, they found that adding omega-3 fatty acids (those found in oily fish and fish oil supplements) produced a dose-dependent decrease in cellular activity linked with cartilage damage. While there is undoubtedly more to learn, it is now clear that stories about eating fish 'to oil your joints' are based on more than hearsay.

Fish oil is extracted from the flesh of oily fish such as herring, mackerel, salmon and trout. It is the best source of the omega-3 fatty acids needed to maintain healthy joints. These fatty acids have the added benefits of discouraging the formation of blood clots and helping to maintain normal blood pressure and cholesterol levels. They also are vital for healthy skin and hair.

Unlike cod liver oil, fish oil contains neither vitamin A nor D, and will not add to a build-up of these nutrients in the liver, which can be toxic in large amounts.

Take fish oil with food, as it may cause nausea when taken on an empty stomach. The usual recommended dose is 1000mg taken three times a day.

COD LIVER OIL

Cod liver oil has been associated with healthy bones and joint mobility since 1922, when it was discovered that a daily dose of cod liver oil prevented rickets, a crippling disease that causes bow legs in children. As the name states, this dietary supplement is derived specifically from the livers of cod fish. Scientists later found that its success in preventing rickets was specifically due to the amount of vitamin D in the oil. Cod liver oil differs from fish oil because it contains substantial amounts of both vitamins A and D, but lower levels of omega-3 fatty acids EPA and DHA (see *Fish Oil*). It is now recognized that the omega-3 fatty acids – which were unknown in 1922 – play an important role in maintaining healthy bones and joints.

A maximum of 3000mg per day is thought to be safe. Higher doses should not be used without a practitioner's supervision because cod liver oil is rich in vitamin A, which can be toxic in large amounts.

Glucosamine sulfate

Glucosamine sulfate is used in the body to build and repair joints, and maintain healthy ligaments, muscles and tendons. It has also been shown to act as an effective non-steroidal anti-inflammatory drug in the treatment of osteoarthritis.

In normal joints a balance exists between the processes that build, or synthesize, cartilage and those that break down or degrade it. In osteoarthritis the balance is tipped in favour of the processes that degrade cartilage. Other anti-inflammatory agents do not restore this balance, and research has shown they can actually add to the negative imbalance. Glucosamine, however, supports the biological processes responsible for synthesis, and so helps restore joint mobility.

Medical treatment for osteoarthritis aims to reduce or stop the degeneration of joint cartilage and control pain and other symptoms associated with this debilitating condition. According to European studies, glucosamine has about the same effect as the NSAID ibuprofen – a common treatment for this form of arthritis – but without the same degree of gastric side effects. Using both reductions in pain and increased movement as indicators, the value of this natural compound was found to be significant.

Some anti-inflammatory drugs reduce pain but inhibit the body's ability to build new joint cartilage. Research strongly suggests that glucosamine actually supports the synthesis of cartilage, and may reduce the inhibition caused by NSAIDs.

The recommended dose is 500–1500mg per day, taken in 500mg doses up to three times a day. Take it with meals to avoid heartburn and indigestion. If you have a sensitive stomach take only one tablet per day. Usually it takes 4–6 weeks before the full effects of glucosamine are felt.

Glucosamine is generally thought to be non-toxic, and at the time this book was written there was no published scientific evidence that it interacted adversely with any medication. However, people sensitive to shellfish may experience mild stomach upset.

Evening primrose oil (epo)

Seed oil from the evening primrose (no relation of the wild primrose) has been used as a food supplement for decades. It is an excellent source of GLA (gammalinoleic acid), an omega-6 fatty acid that some people fail to produce in adequate amounts, and one that has been shown to aid joint mobility, improve skin conditions, and reduce breast tenderness associated with PMS. Certain medications, viral infections, smoking, alcoholic beverages, ageing and excessive amounts of saturated dietary fat all slow the body's production of this vital substance.

When self-supplementing, 3000mg per day is a safe maximum dose. This should be taken separately from fish oil. Note: starflower oil, extracted from the seeds of the borage plant, is frequently taken as a source of GLA. People with certain mental disorders, or those taking tranquillizers, should check with their doctors before using supplements containing GLA.

Which vitamins and minerals are important in preventing and treating arthritis?

Calcium

Calcium makes up about 1.5% of the body's weight, and 99% of this is in bone. It is required for strong bones and teeth, and for normal biological activity in muscles, nerves and blood. Severe deficiency can produce rickets in children, and osteomalacia in adults. It is thought that the development of osteoporosis may be due to a mild deficiency of calcium over a number of years.

It is recommended that adults consume 800mg of calcium per day. The intake for adolescents, nursing mothers and pregnant women should be between 1.0 and 1.4g per day.

Good food sources of calcium include dairy products, canned fish, tofu, dried figs, dark green leafy vegetables and pulses (legumes).

VITAMIN D AND CALCIUM

Vitamin D and calcium are necessary to prevent bone loss and fractures associated with osteoporosis. For many years it was believed that a balanced diet and normal exposure to sunlight provided adequate levels of this important pair of nutrients, but scientists have reconsidered the matter. In the mid-1990s, calcium's role in the prevention of osteoporosis was reviewed and the recommended daily intake for people over 65 was substantially increased from 800mg to 1500mg, or the equivalent of five 240ml/ 8fl oz glasses of milk. Most women in the United States, where the relevant studies took place, consume on average only 600mg each day.

Vitamin D helps the body absorb calcium and transport it to bones. Unfortunately, as we age our digestive systems are less able to absorb calcium; an additional boost of vitamin D helps correct this slow-down. Vitamin D is produced when a compound in the skin absorbs sunlight. As little as 15 minutes exposure per day is adequate to supply normal requirements of the nutrient. However, older people may tend to avoid the sun, and this compounds problems caused by their lowered capacity to absorb the nutrient. Reduced kidney and liver function make matters even worse.

For these reasons, supplements containing vitamin D and calcium are recommended. If you are over 65, or think your diet and sun exposure do not provided adequate levels of these nutrients, experts advise consuming 400 International Units (IU) a day. However, avoid taking excessive amounts of vitamins D. Prolonged intake of 600 micrograms or more a day may have toxic effects, including kidney damage and high blood pressure. Consult your doctor if you are taking digoxin, glycoside medication, or thiazide diuretics before using any supplement containing vitamin D.

Boron and vitamin K also work with calcium to maintain healthy bone structure. When you buy calcium supplements, check to see if these are included in the product.

Vitamin e

There was a time when scientists did not believe that humans required vitamin E for good health. Recent research has shown, however, that this oily substance is a powerful antioxidant with anti-ageing properties. It is thought that vitamin E protects against cardiovascular disease by protecting the HDL cholesterol (sometimes called 'good' cholesterol) from damage by free radicals in the body. This reduces the build-up of atherosclerotic plaques on the walls of blood vessels.

There are other considerable benefits from vitamin E. When taken with vitamin C, vitamin E may also slow the effects of Alzheimer's disease. Damaging free radicals are thought to play a significant role in the development of this debilitating illness, and an increasing number of scientific studies suggest antioxidant vitamins may prevent or slow its progress.

Experts believe it is safe to supplement the diet with 400 IU per day. However, prolonged use of large amounts of vitamin E (more than 1000 IU per day) may cause bleeding in people taking medication to thin the blood.

Vitamin c

People with damaged or painful joints may have an increased need for vitamin C. Heavy smokers, athletes, heavy drinkers and people who are ill or recovering from illness or injury may also wish to supplement their diet with this nutrient.

Recent scientific studies have shown a link between diets rich in vitamin C and lower rates of cardiovascular disease and certain cancers. Vitamin C is also thought to enhance the immune system's response to viral and bacterial infections, and help relieve cold symptoms by acting as a mild antihistamine.

Vitamin C is vital for the production of collagen, found in bone, tendons and skin. Also, in combination with vitamin E, vitamin C is a powerful antioxidant that helps fight any damaging build-up of oxidative free radicals in the body.

According to the National Institutes of Health (NIH), in the United States, a healthy adult should consume 200mg of vitamin C each day.

Only a third of Americans achieve this, and one third consume less than 60mg per day. People eating processed foods as part of westernized diets fail to meet their body's requirements for this crucial vitamin. Happily, the *Eat to Beat Arthritis* Diet provides plenty of fruits and vegetables rich in this vital nutrient.

Experts generally agree that, over the long term, 1500–2000mg of vitamin C a day is safe. Good food sources include red and green peppers, strawberries, kiwi fruit, and citrus fruit.

MAGNESIUM

Magnesium helps maintain healthy bone structure. In Great Britain, tea is a major source of this mineral. Other food sources include avocados, nuts, pulses (legumes) and wholegrains.

SELENIUM

Selenium is a mineral that acts as an anti-inflammatory in the body, and is therefore useful in controlling the symptoms of arthritis. Diets rich in selenium have been linked with lower rates of certain cancers and heart disease. Brazil nuts are the best food source of selenium, but it is also found in liver and other forms of offal, red meat, fish, and wheat grown in soil rich in this mineral. (Note: those suffering from gout should avoid liver and other offal.)

Selenium intake in Great Britain and most of the rest of Europe is very low – half the recommended daily allowance or less. In Finland, the general dietary intake of selenium dropped so low the government considered it a public health hazard, and fertilizers used to grow crops were supplemented with the mineral.

A safe long-term dose is 200 micrograms per day. Do not exceed 700 micrograms, as over time this and higher amounts can become toxic.

What other natural substances hold promise as treatments for arthritis?

CHONDROITIN SULPHATE

Chondroitin is a building substance in cartilage that was once thought to have as much therapeutic value as a dietary supplement as glucosamine. The two were combined in many commercial products. However, research has shown that chondroitin is poorly absorbed by the body, and its value as a supplement appears to be limited. Nutrimax, a company that makes a patented product containing both chondroitin and glucosamine, is funding research to assess its effectiveness.

MSM (METHYLSULFONYLMETHANE)

MSM is found in tiny quantities in every cell in the body. Although we know comparatively little about it, research suggests it is a necessary building block for a number of proteins, including those in muscles, connective tissue and joints.

As it appears to inhibit pain impulses and also act to control inflammation, MSM is one of the newer dietary supplements used to control arthritis. Early work suggests it may be especially useful for people suffering from osteoarthritis.

Testimonials suggest MSM reduces muscle spasms, increases blood flow, and may help repair cartilage. It has also been used to treat lupus and other auto-immune conditions, chronic back pain and to slow the growth of certain cancers.

Ronald M. Laurence, M.D., Ph.D., assistant clinical professor at UCLA School of Medicine, has written a book on this subject (*The Miracle of MSM*, Putnam, 1999). In an interview conducted by www.wholehealth.com, Dr Laurence was asked about the safety of this new supplement. He reportedly said: 'In the thousands of patients I have treated who took 2000mg and more of MSM daily for months and years, I haven't heard of any serious complaints to date.' He continued, 'In fact, I feel comfortable telling people that MSM is safer than water. Remember, though, MSM is a biologically active substance and can sometimes produce side effects, such as skin rash or minor gastrointestinal upset, in some people. If you're on anti-coagulants, you should check with your doctor before taking MSM, because it can occasionally have a blood-thinning effect.'

Dr Laurence recommends taking a combination of MSM and 500mg of glucosamine three times a day, and many patients experience less pain when they use this combination of supplements.

Take with food to minimize gastric upset.

BOSWELLIA

This herb is used as a treatment for arthritis in the traditional medicine of India. It is thought that boswellic acid blocks the action of leukotrines that stimulate an inflammatory response.

CAYENNE CREAM

A topical cream containing capsaicin, the substance in hot peppers that give them their sting, has been found useful in controlling the pain of arthritis. It appears to create a temporary diversion, and inhibits the production of a chemical substance that sends pain messages to the brain.

Use only as recommended on the product.

DMSO (DIMETHYL SULFOXIDE)

An industrial solvent approved by the United States Food and Drug Administration for a bladder disorder known as interstitial cystitis, DMSO was once widely used as an alternative treatment for several forms of arthritis. However, the highly unpleasant smell it caused in users lessened its appeal. It can also have toxic effects in some people. It is now used as a solvent in some products.

NIACINAMIDE

A double-blind study has shown that this form of vitamin B3 is an effective treatment for knee pain. Do not use this supplement without being monitored by your doctor, as high doses (about 3000mg per day) may have serious side effects.

SAME (S-ADENOSYLMETHIOINE)

It has been found that an anti-inflammatory effect similar to that of ibuprofen can be produced by SAMe (pronounced sammy), which is a form of the amino acid methionine. Compared with other non-prescription treatments, this supplement is expensive. It should not be taken by people with manic-depressive illness.

What are some of the alternative therapies used in the treatment of arthritis?

Acupressure – a massage technique in which the fingertips and thumbs apply pressure on specific points along the acupuncture meridians.

Alexander technique – a means of improving movement and posture by the effective and minimal use of muscles.

Aromatherapy – the use of aromatic essential oils to treat pain, inflammation and the underlying cause of many forms of ill-health.

Art therapy – by using art to express their feelings, patients gain relief from pain and the tensions that increase the sensation of pain.

Ayurvedic medicine – an ancient system of holistic healing originating in India. Remedies are based on diet, breathing exercises and yoga.

Bach flower remedies – the use of infusions of different plants to treat health-threatening emotional and physical imbalances.

Chiropractic – a system of manual manipulation of the spine used to relieve pain and illness throughout the body.

Colour therapy – use of colour to affect a person's mental and physical state.

Feldenkrais – the system of yoga, stretching and exercise that improves one's awareness of movement patterns and encourages the proper use of muscle groups.

Herbal medicine – holistic system of medicine based on the healing properties of plants.

Homoeopathy – a healing system based on the belief that minute amounts of substances that cause a symptom in a healthy person will cure that same symptom in one who is ill.

Hydrotherapy – therapy based on the use of different temperatures of water and compresses.

Meditation – a system of spiritual healing in which a person learns to focus their attention on a neutral object and relax.

Microwave therapy – deep heat treatment in which electrodes placed on a person's skin pass electromagnetic waves to deeper parts of the body. The heat created increases blood flow to the area and relieves joint and muscle pain.

Nutritional therapy – the use of specific foods and food supplements to treat illness.

Occupational therapy – a system of care in which trained professionals devise ways for individuals to perform everyday tasks.

Osteopathy – a system of medical practice based on the theory that the loss of physical integrity, or form, causes illness. Treatment involves manipulation of the spine and joints, plus other therapeutic techniques.

Physiotherapy – a system of healing care in which a medical professional uses exercise to help restore movement and strength to the body.

Rolfing – a system of healing based on deep massage intended to realign the body's structure by strengthening the body's connective tissue, thus improving posture and balance.

Shiatsu – a system of treatment similar to acupressure, but here the therapist uses elbows, knees and feet as well as fingers and thumbs when applying pressure to the body's meridian points.

Ultrasound – the use of sound waves to stimulate blood flow to an area of pain.

Yoga – a holistic system of therapy, originating in India, that utilizes breathing, exercises, meditation and relaxation to heal.

Zen – a system of spiritual care, based on Buddhist philosophies, that aims to integrate the mind, body and spirit in achieving a state of total fulfilment.

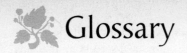# Glossary

This section includes items not mentioned in this book, but which may be of interest to the reader.

Acute disease: A short, severe illness.

Allergens: Substances that cause allergies.

Allergy: An abnormal immune response to harmless substances causing one or more of the following symptoms: itching (especially around the mouth), hay fever (sneezing), rash and swelling. Extreme reactions may lead to bronchospasm, anaphylactic shock and death.

Amaranth: A grain discovered in ancient caves in Mexico. It is high in the amino acid lysine, and is favoured by some nutritional therapists for its healing properties. It is usually available in health food stores.

Amino acids: The basic building blocks for proteins. There are 20 amino acids in the human body, and most can be manufactured by it. However, there are eight amino acids that must be supplied by food. These are tryptophane, isoleucine, leucine, lysine, threonine, methionine, phenalanine and valine. Two other amino acids (histidine and arginine) can be made in the adult body, but not that of young children, and are therefore known as 'semi-essential' amino acids.

Dietary protein should include all the essential amino acids, because the absence of any one acid can cause protein deficiency. Including meat in your diet eliminates this possibility. Protein supplied by plant sources, such as grains and pulses (legumes), does not contain the full complement of amino acids: some are missing in grains, while others are missing in pulses. If you are a vegetarian, you should therefore mix grains and pulses in the same meal.

Two ancient grains from South America, quinoa and amaranth, are excellent plant protein sources because they both contain all the amino acids required for good health.

ANA (antinuclear antibody) test: A means of determining if the body is producing antibodies that cause auto-immune disorders by attacking the nuclei of healthy cells in connective tissue.

Analgesic: Any medication that controls pain.

Ankylosing spondylitis: A form of rheumatic arthritis affecting the spine and lower back.

Antibody: A protein produced by white blood cells in response to a specific substance, or *antigen*. The antibody binds itself to the antigen and neutralizes it.

Antigen: Any substance introduced into the body that stimulates the production of antibodies by the immune system. (See *Immune system*.)

Antioxidant: A substance that is able to block the harmful effects of excessive free radicals produced during the process of oxidation. Vitamins E and C are examples of powerful natural antioxidants. (See *Free radicals*.)

Atrophy: Wasting away of a body part or tissue. Muscles, for example, atrophy following long periods of inactivity.

Auto-antibodies: Antibodies that react to and destroy normal body cells and tissues, thus causing illness. (See *Auto-immune disease*.)

Auto-immune disease: Any abnormal condition arising when a person's immune system produces antibodies that attack normal tissues. Examples are rheumatoid arthritis, SLE (*Systemic lupus erythematosus*), auto-immune infertility, diabetes mellitus type 1, and auto-immune haemolytic anaemia.

Benign illness: A relatively mild form of a disease; non-life threatening.

Bone marrow: The spongy soft tissue found in the cavities of bones. Two forms exist: yellow bone marrow, which mostly consists of connective tissue and fat; and red bone marrow, which is the source of most blood cells including red blood cells, stem cells and platelets. In adults, red marrow is found in the collarbones, breastbone, ribs, spine, pelvis, shoulder blades and bones of the skull.

Bursa: A sac-like structure, lined with cells that secrete a lubricating fluid. It serves as a cushion between bones, muscles and tendons, and helps them glide over one another.

Bursitis: Inflammation of a *bursa*. Examples are 'frozen shoulder', 'student's elbow' and 'housemaid's knee'.

Carbohydrates: The components of food that are its primary source of energy. About 50 per cent of calories in a healthy diet come from carbohydrates. These are made up of chains of molecules of different building blocks, or 'sugars'. These can be simple in form, or complex.

Simple sugars are sweet, and add enjoyment to many of the foods we eat. When used in purified form – such as table sugar – simple sugars have little nutritional value other than as a source of fast energy; when this energy is excessive, and not burned off through exercise, it is stored in the body as fat. Simple sugars – like that used on cereal or in sweets – can cause the blood sugar level to fluctuate, sometimes causing mood swings.

By contrast, long chain sugars (polysaccharides, also known as starches) release their energy slowly into the body, and help keep blood sugar levels within healthy limits.

Some complex carbohydrates we eat are not digested by the human body, and pass unused through the digestive system. Known as 'dietary fibre', these complex carbohydrates form a vital part of nature's internal cleansing process.

Cartilage: A flexible, tough form of connective tissue. For arthritis sufferers, the most important cartilage is found at the ends of bones, where it acts as a shock absorber during motion. In osteoarthritis, cartilage is slowly destroyed through wear and tear (see *osteoarthritis*). Cartilage also forms structural parts of the body, including the ears and nose.

Cell: The smallest complete unit in the body, consisting of a membrane, nucleus, cell fluid and small structures called organelles. Cells are the metabolic engines of life.

Chronic illness: A lingering illness – the opposite of *acute*.

Chronic degenerative diseases: Illnesses associated with the processes of ageing and the slow deterioration of body structures.

Collagen: The main protein component of connective tissue. Collagen is damaged during many inflammatory illnesses, including rheumatoid arthritis.

Connective tissue: Structural tissue that holds parts of the body together and gives it form. For example, blood vessels and bone have shape because of connective tissue. Cartilage and tendons are forms of connective tissue.

Contracture: Crippling joint deformity resulting in the loss of motion and shrinking of surrounding tissues.

Elimination diet: The process of identifying foods which cause sensitive or allergic reactions. Two methods commonly used are either to introduce foods one at a time and watch for symptoms; or to eliminate individual foods until a food sensitivity or allergic reaction clears.

Endorphins: Natural substances in the brain that stop pain. Exercise, chocolate, chillies and honey all increase endorphin levels.

Enzymes: Protein catalysts produced by cells that support the biological processes of life without changing their own structure.

ESR (erythrocyte sedimentation rate): A clinical test that measures the rate at which red blood cells settle to the bottom of a test tube. A high ESR indicates an inflammatory disease, such as rheumatoid arthritis.

Essential fatty acids: A group of fats required by the human body for normal health. These fats cannot be manufactured by the human body, and must be obtained from food, or consumed as dietary supplements. Two forms exist, each having its own biological structure and significance; these are omega-3 and omega-6 fatty acids.

Omega-3 fatty acids help prevent heart disease and maintain healthy joints. Oily fish are excellent sources of these substances.

Linolenic acid, the basic omega-3 fatty acid, is most commonly obtained from oily fish, some nuts, and certain green foods. This molecule is metabolized by the body to form *DHA* and *EPA*. Under certain circumstances (illness, stress, using excessive amounts of alcohol, smoking and taking certain medications) the body fails to metabolize adequate amounts of linolenic acid. In these cases DHA- and EPA-rich supplements are helpful. The metabolic process responsible for the first step in the conversion of both linoleic and linolenic acid is the same and, therefore, there is competition between these nutrients.

Omega-6 fatty acids are important structural parts of normal cell membranes and small hormone substances (prostaglandins) that regulate body functions. Plant seed oils are good sources of these nutrients.

Linoleic acid, the basic omega-6 fatty acid, is most commonly consumed as part of seed and nut oils. This molecule is metabolized by the body to form gamma-linolenic acid (GLA), which are then further converted into other fatty acids vital for good health. Under certain circumstances (illness, stress, using excessive amounts of alcohol, smoking, and taking certain medications) the body fails to metabolize adequate amounts of linoleic acid. In these cases, GLA-rich supplements are necessary.

Three important metabolites of essential fatty acids are:

GLA (*gamma-linolenic acid*): An omega-6 fatty acid found useful in treating a number of conditions, including premenstrual tension. It is produced by the body during the metabolism of linoleic acid.

DHA (*docosahexaenoic acid*): An omega-3 essential fatty acid that has been shown to have a positive effect on inflammation. It is also important for normal brain function.

EPA (*eicosapentaenoic acid*): An omega-3 essential fatty acid shown to have a positive effect on inflammation. It is important for a normal central nervous system.

When used as dietary supplements, omega-3 and omega-6 fatty acids should be taken at different times and always with food.

Evening primrose oil: An oil extracted from the seeds of an ancient healing plant found in North America, which is now used as the major source of *GLA*.

Fat: An important source of energy and building material for a healthy body, dietary fat is also the sole source of essential nutrients such as vitamins D and E, and the essential fatty acids (see *Essential fatty acids*). As part of a normal healthy diet, fat should provide about one-third of the total calories consumed. The type of fat we eat is important to our health. Saturated fat, like that found in red meat and dairy products, should make up no more that 10 per cent of our total fat intake. Many vegetarians are unaware that their diet is high in saturated fat due to their dependence on dairy products for protein.

Most of the fat in a healthy diet should be monounsaturated, like that found in olive oil and avocados.

Polyunsaturated fats are the most biologically beneficial of the fats, and should make up about 20 per cent of total intake. Vitamin E is needed to protect these fats against oxidation. Good food sources include wheatgerm oil, safflower oil, sunflower oil and almonds.

Remember: processing foods destroys the delicate structure of polyunsaturated fatty acids and removes their biological benefits.

Fish oil (marine oil): Oils extracted from the bodies of oily fish, such as mackerel, herring and salmon. Fish oil is not the same as cod liver oil, which is extracted from the livers of fish. Pure fish oil naturally contains a higher concentration of the essential fatty acids DHA and EPA, but contains less vitamins A and D than oil extracted from fish livers.

Remember: vitamin A levels in fish liver oil are high, and excessive amounts can be toxic.

Flare: A hot, red area often seen over, or around, an arthritic joint. A sign of inflammation.

Free radical: A molecule of a substance that has lost part of its electrical charge through the process of oxidation. Free radicals are part of normal chemical processes in the body; in excess, however, they are a contributing cause in many degenerative illnesses, including rheumatoid arthritis. (See *Antioxidant*.)

Gluten: A form of protein found in wheat, rye and barley that may cause food sensitivity, including coeliac disease. Oats contain a substance with properties similar to gluten.

Gluten is not used by the human body, and is therefore not a necessary part of a healthy diet. However, because its presence enhances the texture and appearance of many foods, it is frequently added to processed foods.

Gout: A type of arthritis caused by crystals of uric acid forming in joints. Symptoms are inflammation, swelling and acute pain. Gout affects more men than women, and frequently occurs in a big toe. (See *Uric acid*.)

Gram (g): A measure of weight equal to one thousandth of a kilogram.

Immune system: The combination of organs and cells in the body that work to protect the body from invasion by bacteria, fungi and viruses.

Inflammation/Inflammatory response: Localized pain, heat, redness and swelling that develop as part of an immune response. Increased blood flow, the concentration of fluid in an area, and the accumulation of white blood cells are involved. Inflammation is normally observed following an infection, although it also occurs under abnormal conditions, such as an *auto-immune* reaction.

Isoflavins: Natural plant compounds. Populations enjoying diets rich in these substances have lower risks of heart disease, certain cancers and menopausal symptoms. Good food sources are soya products, such as tofu, and linseed. The western diet is low in isoflavins.

Joint: A place where two bones meet. There are several types of joints: some are mobile, like those in the arms and legs, and others are immobile, such as those between the bones of the skull.

Joint capsule: See *Synovial sac*.

Juvenile rheumatoid arthritis: A chronic and crippling form of arthritis seen in children.

Leukotrines: Hormone-like substances, derived from omega-6 essential fatty acids, that play a role in inflammation.

Ligaments: Strap-like fibres attached to bones that help maintain their normal alignment.

Marine oils: See *Fish oil*.

Metabolism: The continuous chain of chemical reactions that take place in the living body. Food and tissues are broken down (*catabolism*), while new substances are built-up for use in the production of energy, or to replace parts of body cells and cell products (*anabolism*).

Microgram (ug): A measure of weight equal to one millionth of a gram.

Milligram (mg): A measure of weight equal to one thousandth of a gram.

Molecule: The smallest existing amount of any chemical compound that maintains the characteristic of that substance.

Nodules: Areas of confined inflammation that commonly appear under the skin of people suffering from rheumatoid arthritis.

NSAIDs: Non-steroidal anti-inflammatory drugs used to suppress pain and inflammation. Aspirin and ibuprofen are examples.
   Remember: NSAIDs inhibit the production of prostaglandins in the lining of the stomach and may encourage the formation of ulcers.

Nutrition: The balance of basic substances that the body requires from food to enable it to maintain normal growth and good health. Well-balanced nutrition protects the body, whereas poor nutrition encourages disease. Poor nutrition can cause illness by itself, through dietary deficiency, or it can increase the possibility of illness by damaging the immune system and reducing the disease-resistance of body tissues.

Osteoarthritis (also known as *degenerative joint disease*): Damage to joints that affects the cartilage pads at the ends of bones. Cartilage may fray, wear, or even wear away entirely. The onset of osteoarthritis frequently follows damage or prolonged stress on a joint.

Osteoporosis: The loss of bone mass and strength that increases the risk of fractures. Believed by many to be a natural part of ageing, osteoporosis is most common in post-menopausal women, elderly men and people who do not consume adequate quantities of calcium in their diet.

Pauciarticular: Arthritis affecting four or fewer joints.

Polyarticular: Arthritis affecting five or more joints.

Prostaglandins: Substances in the body with hormone-like activity. Essential fatty acids make up a part of their molecular structure. Certain prostaglandins cause the symptoms of inflammation.

Proteins: One of the four major components of food (protein, carbohydrate, fat and water) that are needed for the normal structure and activity of all cells in the body. Proteins are complex molecules made up of basic building blocks called *amino acids*. Protein should provide 10–15 per cent of the total calories in a healthy diet.

Purines: Natural substances found in anchovies, asparagus, cauliflower, game, mushrooms, offal (liver, kidneys and heart), peas, poultry, pulses (beans, chickpeas, lentils), sardines, shellfish and spinach. These foods can increase the level of uric acid in the blood, thus making it more likely to precipitate in joints and soft tissues, such as the kidneys. (See *Uric acid*.)

People suffering from gout should avoid foods high in purines.

Range of motion (ROM): The extent to which a joint can progress through its normal movements. ROM exercises are important in arthritis because they increase or maintain movement and flexibility of muscles, joint, ligaments and tendons.

Rheumatism: A general term used to describe inflammatory conditions of the skeleton and muscles. Also used as a general term to describe aches and pains.

Acute rheumatism, also known as rheumatic fever, most frequently occurs in childhood following a streptococcal throat infection. Symptoms include polyarthritis of the larger joints, fever, and inflammation of the heart, which can result in long-term consequences. Treatment with penicillin is effective.

Rheumatoid arthritis: A chronic inflammation of joint linings (synovial linings) that causes pain, swelling and stiffness. Loss of joint function may occur.

Rheumatoid factor (*RF*): An antibody found in the blood of most people suffering from rheumatoid arthritis.

Quinoa: Called the mother grain by the Incas, quinoa is actually a distant relative of the beet family, and is not really a grain but a fruit. It is nutritionally valuable as it contains all eight essential amino acids, in perfect balance. It is available in health food stores.

Serous membrane: The thin layer of cells that form a lining over all the closed surfaces of the body, including the joints. They secrete a watery fluid that serves as a lubricant between moving body parts.

Serum: The clear fluid that separates from blood when it clots.

Spurs: The bony outcrops that occur within joints afflicted by osteoarthritis.

Sugars: See *Carbohydrates*.

Synovial fluid: Fluid found in synovial sacs surrounding joints.

Synovial sac: The fibrous capsule encasing the contents of a joint.

Tendons: Cords of tough fibrous tissue that connect muscles to bone.

Uric acid: A waste product from the metabolism of proteins. Under normal conditions this relatively insoluble substance is released into the blood, carried to the kidneys, and excreted in the urine. Under abnormal circumstances – such as the long-term use of certain medications – the kidneys fail to excrete adequate amounts of uric acid, which remains in the blood. As the level rises, it crystallizes out of the blood and forms deposits in various tissues around the body, including the joints. Gout can be extremely painful and although there are drugs that can help reduce the problem, dietary measures to control the amount and type of protein eaten are an important part of any treatment programme. (See *Gout*.)

Vitamins: A group of nutrients that cannot be manufactured by the human body, but are absolutely essential for specific metabolic activities in living tissue. Absence of one or more vitamins over time leads to deficiency diseases, such as scurvy (vitamin C deficiency).

There are two types of vitamins: those soluble in water (vitamin C and all the B vitamins are examples), and those vitamins that are soluble in oil (such as vitamins A, E and D).

The body's demand for individual vitamins varies with age, physical condition and lifestyle. Smoking, for example, greatly increases the need for vitamin C. Menstrual bleeding and childbirth increase the need for iron.

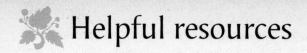# Helpful resources

SELECTED READING

A Doctor's Proven New Home Cure for Arthritis, Giraud W. Campbell D.O., Thorsons, London. 1989.

8 Weeks to Optimum Health, Andrew Weil, M.D., Little, Brown and Company, London. 1997.

Clear Body Clear Mind: How to be Healthy in a Polluted World, Leon Chaitow, Gaia Books Ltd., London. 1990.

The Everyday Wheat-free and Gluten-free Cookbook, Michelle Berriedale-Johnson, Grub Street, London. 1998.

The Fats We Need to Eat, Jeannette Ewin PhD., Thorsons, London. 1995.

The Green Pharmacy, James A. Duke, Ph.D., Rodale Press, Emmaus, Pennsylvania. 1997.

Healing with Whole Food: Oriental Traditions and Modern Nutrition, Paul Pitchford, North Atlantic Books, Berkeley, California. 1993.

USEFUL ADDRESSES

All addresses were correct at the time of going to press. Do remember, however, that website addresses (usually those not attached to established organisations) tend to change.

The United States
National Institute of Arthritis and Musculoskeletal and Skin Diseases (NIAMS)
National Institutes of Health
Bethesda, Maryland
USA

United Kingdom
The Arthritic Association
1st Floor Suite
2 Hyde Gardens
Eastbourne BN21 4PN
Telephone (01323) 416550
www.arthriticassociation.org.uk

Arthritis Care (Help line)
18 Stephenson Way
London NW1 2HD
(020) 7916 1500
www.arthritiscare.org.uk

The Institute for Optimum Nutrition
Blades Court
Deodar Road
London SW15 2NU
Telephone: (020) 8877 9993
www.ion.ac.uk

National Osteoporosis Society
P.O. Box 10
Radstock
Bath
BA3 3YB
(01761) 471771
www.nos.org.uk

**Arthritis Research Campaign,
Medical Research Charity**
Copeman House
St Mary's Court
Mary's Gate
Chesterfield
S41 7TD
(01246) 558033
www.arc.org.uk

Australia
Australian Nutrition Foundation
1–3 Derwent Street
Glebe
NSW 2037
Telephone: 02 9552 3081

OTHER USEFUL WEBSITES
Arthritis
Arthritis Information Resources –
www.pslgroup.com/arthritis.htm

The Arthritis Society of Canada –
www.arthritis.ca

Arthritis Victoria –
www.arthritisvic.org.au

National Institute of Arthritis and
Musculoskeletal and Skin Diseases,
National Institutes of Health –
www.nih.gov/niams

Arthritis News Break Newsletter –
www.hsc.missouri.edu/~arthritis/an
btp.html

www.arthritiswebsite.com

General medical information
American Academy of Family
Physicians www.aafp.org/healthinfo

www.bbc.co.uk/health

www.britannica.com (One of the
best free websites available. Provides
links to other sites.)

www.docguide.com

www.healthy.net

www.mayohealth.org

www.netdoctor.co.uk

www.webmd.com

www.wholehealth.com

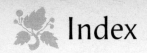

Index